FREUD
AND
MODERN
PSYCHOLOGY

VOLUME 2: THE EMOTIONAL BASIS
OF HUMAN BEHAVIOR

EMOTIONS, PERSONALITY, AND PSYCHOTHERAPY

Series Editors
Carroll E. Izard, *University of Delaware, Newark, Delaware*
and
Jerome L. Singer, *Yale University, New Haven, Connecticut*

HUMAN EMOTIONS
   Carroll E. Izard

THE PERSONAL EXPERIENCE OF TIME
   Bernard S. Gorman and Alden E. Wessman

THE STREAM OF CONSCIOUSNESS: Scientific Investigation into the
Flow of Human Experience
   Kenneth S. Pope and Jerome L. Singer, eds.

THE POWER OF HUMAN IMAGINATION: New Methods
in Psychotherapy
   Jerome L. Singer and Kenneth S. Pope, eds.

EMOTIONS IN PERSONALITY AND PSYCHOPATHOLOGY
   Carroll E. Izard, ed.

FREUD AND MODERN PSYCHOLOGY, Volume 1: The Emotional
Basis of Mental Illness
   Helen Block Lewis

FREUD AND MODERN PSYCHOLOGY, Volume 2: The Emotional
Basis of Human Behavior
   Helen Block Lewis

GUIDED AFFECTIVE IMAGERY WITH CHILDREN AND ADOLESCENTS
   Hanscarl Leuner, Günther Horn, and Edda Klessmann

A Continuation Order Plan is available for this series. A continuation order will bring delivery of each new volume immediately upon publication. Volumes are billed only upon actual shipment. For further information please contact the publisher.

FREUD

AND

MODERN

PSYCHOLOGY

VOLUME 2: THE EMOTIONAL BASIS
OF HUMAN BEHAVIOR

HELEN BLOCK LEWIS

Yale University
New Haven, Connecticut

PLENUM PRESS · NEW YORK AND LONDON

Library of Congress Cataloging in Publication Data

Lewis, Helen B.
    Freud and modern psychology.

    (Emotions, personality, and psychotherapy)
    Includes bibliographies and indexes.
    Contents: v. 1. The emotional basis of mental illness—v. 2. The emotional basis of
human behavior.
    1. Psychology, Pathological. 2. Emotions. 3. Interpersonal relations. 4. Freud, Sigmund,
1856–1939. 5. Psychoanalysis. I. Title. II. Series.
RC454.L48   616.89'001'9   80-20937
ISBN 0-306-40525-3 (v. 1)
ISBN 0-306-41329-9 (v. 2)

©1983 Plenum Press, New York
A Division of Plenum Publishing Corporation
233 Spring Street, New York, N.Y. 10013

Printed in the United States of America

Preface

Freud's discovery of an emotional basis for mental illness led him to pursue the emotional basis of human behavior in general. This pursuit led him to undertake observational studies of dreams (1900), everyday mistakes (1901), sexuality (1905b), character formation (1908, 1931), jokes (1905a), and the origin of guilt (1913). Volume 2 of *Freud and Modern Psychology* examines the texts of each of these major writings in general psychology, continuing to explore the contradiction between Freud's observations about the power of emotions and his narrow theoretical formulations about human behavior. Volume 2 also reviews the remarkable power of the uniquely moral emotions of shame and guilt not only to create psychiatric symptoms, as discussed in Volume 1, but to infiltrate our nightly dreams, create everyday parapraxes, influence the development of sexuality, specify the emotional release in jokes, shape personality, and "create" human culture.

As we saw in Volume 1, we shall see again in Volume 2 that Freud's theoretical difficulties arose from the absence of a viable theory of human nature as cultural, that is, social by biological origin. In a theoretical framework based on the cultural nature of human nature, the emotions and the social cohesion are reciprocally related to each other. The emotions are the means of the social cohesion which, in turn, is the means by which the emotions, including shame and guilt, are formed in infancy. Volume 2 also shows clearly how (still) prevailing androcentric attitudes influenced Freud's neglect of the infant–caretaker affectional system in his theorizing, as contrasted to his observations.

It is a pleasure to acknowledge the assistance of the Behavioral Science Publications Fund of Yale University in the preparation of the manuscript of Volume 2. Carroll Izard has again been a very helpful editor. Frances DeGrenier has my gratitude for her patience and skill with the word processor. As always, my husband, Naphtali Lewis, has been an unfailing source of support.

Contents

CHAPTER 1

The Interpretation of Dreams
The Problem of Emotions in Dreaming

Freud's main point about dreams was expressed in the title of his book: Dreams can be interpreted in a way that makes emotional sense even though they may appear to be meaningless and to be about trivial events. Nowhere in Freud's work, however, is the contradiction between his insights about the power of emotions and his theoretical neglect of them clearer than in his work on dreams. As Richard Jones (1974) points out, there are, for example, really two distinct books in Freud's *The Interpretation of Dreams* (1900). One book, in six chapters, is about the *interpretation* of dreams into their emotional content. The last chapter (Chapter 7) of *The Interpretation of Dreams* is another book on the *theory* of dreams, in which emotions are hardly mentioned.

The discrepancy between Freud's clinical insights and his theory has also become apparent as a result of the almost accidental discovery, in 1953, of the hitherto unknown rapid eye movement state (REMS) in which dreaming takes place (Aserinsky & Kleitman, 1953). The physiologists' discovery that dreaming occurs roughly four times a night regardless of a person's emotional state was a blow to the specifics of Freud's theory of dream instigation. It was also, however, a roundabout confirmation of his clinical insight that dreaming, mental illness, and emotional life are somehow closely connected. The biochemical triggers that have been implicated in the functioning of the REMS are the very same substances implicated in the biochemistry of mental illness:

serotonin, acetylcholine, norepinephrine, to name a few of the prominent substances. The new biology and psychology of dreaming during
the REMS is one of the most important scientific discoveries of the
twentieth century because it allows new hope that knowledge of the
REMS will somehow unravel the connection between emotional states
and mental illness.

Eye movements during sleep and dreams had been observed as
early as 1867 by a psychiatrist named Griesinger (cited by Snyder, 1967).
Although these and similar observations were reported several times by
different observers over the next decades, they were never systematically pursued. But in 1953, because of Freud's intervening work, the
finding that eye movements occur during regularly recurring intervals of
natural sleep and that they signal dreaming, was the start of an enor-
mously productive era of dream research, thus illustrating once again
the zigzag course of the history of ideas.

Freud always regarded *The Interpretation of Dreams* (1900) as his most
important book. In the preface of the third edition of it, he wrote that
"insight such as this falls to one's lot but once in a lifetime." Although
interest in Freud's interpretation of dreaming was slow in developing—
only 351 copies of the book were sold during the first 6 years after
publication—its impact when it finally gained attention was enormous.
For example, the "stream of consciousness" (a phrase actually coined by
William James) entered the modern novel. Mann, Joyce, Woolf, Kafka,
Faulkner, and Dreiser are a few of the twentieth-century novelists
whose art was deepened by Freud's insight into dreams. In his tribute to
Freud, Mann (cited by Puner, 1978) put it this way: "A blithe scepticism
has come into the world, a mistrust which unmasks all the schemes and
subterfuges of our own souls." Dreiser, similarly, spoke of the "light
that he has thrown on the human mind . . . at once colossal and
beautiful!"

One example will illustrate the relation between the Freudian study
of dreams and the study of the modern psychological novel. Some years
ago my colleagues and I obtained the hypnagogic reveries and dreams of
people who had seen an emotionally charged film before going to sleep
(Bertini, Lewis, & Witkin, 1964). One film in the series shows a mother
monkey trying to revive her dead baby and then beginning to eat it. In
the course of reverie (right before the sounds of snoring were recorded
on the tape), one subject's horror thoughts about the cannibal mother
and her dead baby changed into thoughts and images of a frog—a
"blue-green frog with dark gray spots" in a surrounding scene that was
quite idyllic: "stones at the bottom of a clear blue pool," "a blue water-
fall," and "a pattern of leaves and then it disappears." In his discussion

of the modern psychological novel, Leon Edel (1964) comments on the content of this reverie, which offers fitful glimpses into the stream of consciousness. Edel makes the point that monitoring a stream of consciousness gives us the raw data of creative writing, which are then "washed out through a sieve, to be used in fiction, as prospectors wash away earth to find gold." Writers have surely always done this, but since *The Interpretation of Dreams* the stream of consciousness has been explicitly honored and even cultivated. "Primary-process" transformations of mingled empathy and disgust are symbolically represented in the hypnagogic reverie that Edel cites. As Edel puts it:

> This passage from life is illuminating; and art could improve it without diminishing its authenticity. For what Joyce and Faulkner and Mrs. Woolf have done—and Tolstoy before them—has been simply to infuse their personal poetry into the often turgid data of consciousness. . . . one of the limitations of Joyce has been that he gloried a little too much in turgidity; but we can imagine how Faulkner might use the "blue waterfall" in this passage or the "stones at the bottom of a clear blue pool." And we know what delicate moments of perception Virginia Woolf would find in a "pattern of leaves and then it disappears" or the "blue-green frog with dark gray spots." . . . mysterious is the dialectic of the mind; and it requires the mysterious process of poetry—as our "subjective" novelists have shown— to render it. (p. 153)

FREUD'S INTERPRETATION OF DREAMS

The present chapter will be devoted to an exposition of the first six chapters of *The Interpretation of Dreams* and to an account of how Freud's method of dream interpretation (as distinct from his theory of dreams) has illuminated our understanding of what happens to people's forbidden feelings. Our exposition will be aided by reference to the paper, *On Dreams* (1901a), Freud's own outline of his work. Reviewing Freud's clinical insights about dreams is of particular importance because the disconfirmation of his theory of dreaming has been an impetus, especially among academic psychologists, to neglect his method of interpreting the dream's representations of strangulated affect. As we shall see, the observations that Freud made about the emotional meaning of dreams have been widely confirmed, even in cross-cultural studies.

Freud opens his treatise boldly with the following statement:

> In the pages that follow I shall bring forward proof that there is a psychological technique which makes it possible to interpret dreams, and that, if that procedure is employed, every dream reveals itself as a psychical structure which has a meaning and which can be inserted at an assignable point in the

mental activities of waking life. I shall further endeavor to elucidate the processes to which the strangeness and obscurity of dreams are due and to deduce from those processes the nature of the psychical forces by whose concurrent or mutually opposing action dreams are generated. (p. 1)

It is worth noting that, in this forthright opening statement, Freud speaks of two separate issues: the interpretation or emotional meaning of dream content, and a theory of the genesis of dreams. Even though the thesis of his book is that dreams are interpretable into their emotional meaning, he omits the word "emotional," using only the ambiguous term "meaning," which by itself has a neutral or ideational connotation, and speaks of "psychical structure" or "psychical forces."

Let us anticipate our story for a moment to see how Freud sounds when he is talking about the forbidden feelings that a dream expresses. I am now quoting from a section on "affect in dreams," toward the end of the book. He uses an example from waking life to demonstrate how affects work.

There is a person of my acquaintance whom I hate, so that I have a lively inclination to feel glad if anything goes wrong with him. But the moral side of my nature will not give way to this impulse. I do not dare to express a wish that he should be unlucky, and if he meets with some undeserved misfortune, I suppress my satisfaction at it and force myself to manifestations and thoughts of regret. Everyone must have found himself in this situation at some time or other. What now happens, however, is that the hated person, by a piece of misconduct of his own, involves himself in some unpleasantness; when that happens I may give free rein to my satisfaction that he has met a just punishment and in this I find myself in agreement with many other people who are impartial. I may observe, however, that my satisfaction seems more intense than that of these other people; it has received an accession from the source of my hatred which till then had been prevented from producing its affect, but in the altered circumstances is no longer hindered from doing so. (p. 478)

Freud is thus clearly talking about feelings of hatred, of guilt, and of righteous indignation. He is suggesting that when the last of these feelings is undiluted by compassion there are likely to be unconscious sources of hatred operating underneath the righteous attitude.

Let us also look at the simile by which he describes the forbidding agency (guilt and shame) in dreams. It is

as though (Freud's italics) one person who was dependent upon a second person had to make a remark which was bound to be disagreeable in the ears of this second one; and it is on the basis of this simile that we have arrived at the concepts of dream-distortion and dream censorship. (p. 677)

In these instances, Freud is clearly referring to an interaction between people which can also take place internally. And, very specifically, he is referring to experiences in which we either confront guilt and shame or turn away from them so that we are not aware of our troubled personal relationships. But when it comes to speculating or theorizing about dreams, Freud thinks not in terms of the feelings of guilt and shame which are at issue, but in terms of impulses, ideas, quantities of excitation and the like.

Before embarking on his main task, Freud, in true scholarly fashion, offers his readers a "review of the scientific literature" on dreams. He tells us, moreover, that he found this review difficult to write because "in spite of many thousands of years of effort, the scientific understanding of dreams has made very little advance" (p. 1). What Freud does with his literature review, therefore, is to gather from it previous observations about the many problems and questions that had aroused his curiosity. Do dreams continue the thoughts we have in waking life? Do dreams deal with immediately preceding events or with forgotten memories? What is the role of somatic stimuli in dreams? Do dreams really only come from "indigestion," or do they have a more emotionally meaningful stimulus? Why are dreams so readily forgotten? Why do they, as Freud says, "melt away"? What makes dream experiences so strange? Are they strange because the mind is just "playing" in sleep, or because their strangeness disguises their meaning? Why are dreams hallucinatory experiences, so unlike the conceptual forms in which thinking takes place during the day? Do dreams reflect the moral life of the dreamer, or "do the dictates of morality have no place in dreams" (p. 66)? What is the function of dreaming? Or do dreams have psychological function? Are they just meaningless or superfluous phenomena of physiological changes occurring during sleep? And, finally, is there any relationship between dreams and mental illness?

The questions that Freud raised at the outset of his book thus form a clear progression leading from the apparently fragile connections between dreams and waking life to the connections between dreams and moral dilemmas, and thence to the connection between dreams and mental illness.

By the end of his book, Freud was able to show that dreams do continue the thoughts of waking life; that they deal with both immediate events and forgotten memories; that they incorporate somatic stimuli but connect them with important feelings; that they are readily forgotten *because* they are emotionally important; that they are strange and hallucinatory because they represent our censored feelings in a special form of affective thinking which he called "primary process." He was also able to state a hypothesis about one of the dream's functions: It is to prevent our waking up; in this sense, dreams are the "guardians of sleep."

(Freud was aware how little was actually known about sleep. But he was a good enough physiologist to suspect that sleep was an organismic need.) The hypothesis that dreams are the guardians of sleep also served to distinguish between dreams and neurotic symptoms. Although the latter are similar in their "primary-process" formation, they occur under very different conditions.

In his review of the literature on the function of dreaming, Freud is particularly sympathetic to the work of a philosopher named Scherner, who had theorized that dreams are "productive" works of the mind when it is freed from the constraints of reason during sleep. The imaginative capacities of the mind then have full sway, gaining in "pliancy, agility and versatility" (p. 84). Defending Scherner's notion that the ego's imaginative capacities are released in sleep, Freud wrote: "It may honestly be said that in attempting to explain dreams it is not easy to avoid being fantastic. Ganglion cells can be fantastic too" (p. 87). It is worth noting, in passing, that Scherner's views are very similar to the views later espoused by Jung and still later by Fromm, both former students of Freud. The bitter opposition between Freud and his students, however, was to come later. In 1900, Freud still described Scherner's views with considerable admiration for their grasp of dream symbolism.

On the question of the relationship between dreams and mental illness, Freud found himself in opposition to the "medical view" that dreams and psychosis are alike in being senseless and meaningless states. He cites Griesinger (whose observations about eye movements in dreaming have been mentioned above) as an authority for the view that dreams and mental illness are alike in being *"fulfillments of wishes"* (Freud's italics). The contrast, Freud emphasizes, is between a view of dreaming as the consequence of psychic insufficiency and as the consequence of unfulfilled longings. But it should be noted that in his discussion of the problems and issues in understanding dreams, he is open to many-sided answers. The lowered efficiency of thought during sleep may play a part; "indigestion" or other "external" stimuli may be incorporated in dreams. Even his exposition of dream theory in Chapter 7 is very tentatively phrased; only later on did the answers to questions about dreaming become rigidified by Freud himself and by his faithful followers.

Freud opens the chapter that follows his literature survey by offering a dream of his own as an example of how to interpret. (The dream he offers is the now-famous "Irma" dream, since reinterpreted by Erik Erikson, 1954.) But before plunging into its text and interpretation, Freud raises still another issue: whether dreams should be interpreted as a whole, or by analyzing the text element by element. This issue is perhaps the most notorious example of a question to which there later developed an "orthodox" answer—namely, that *only* breakdown by elements is safe—even though Freud's interpretation of his Irma dream clearly makes use of *both* holistic and analytical treatments of the text.

This difference between symbolic dream interpretation by grasping the total meaning of a dream—"the way one grasps similarities," as Aristotle had suggested—and dream interpretation by "decoding" elements, rests on a difference in approach to the manifest text. Symbolic interpretation makes direct use of the manifest dream, without any decoding. Decoding, of course, was Freud's unique discovery. It was the discovery he made when he first unraveled neurotic symptoms by the method of free association. The passage in which Freud makes the connection between his work on dreams and his prior work with patients is important enough to quote extensively:

> I have been engaged for many years (with a therapeutic aim in view) in unravelling certain psychopathological structures—hysterical phobias, obsessional ideas, and so on. I have been doing so, in fact, ever since I learnt from an important communication by Josef Breuer that as regards these structures (which are looked on as pathological symptoms) unravelling them coincides with removing them (cf. Breuer & Freud, 1895). If a pathological idea of this sort can be traced back to the elements in a patient's life from which it originated, it simultaneously crumbles away and the patient is freed from it. . . . It was in the course of these psycho-analytic studies that I came upon dream-interpretation. My patients were pledged to communicate to me every idea or thought that occurred to them in connection with some particular subject; amongst other things they told me their dreams and so taught me that a dream can be inserted into the psychical chain that has to be traced backwards in the memory from a pathological idea. It was then only a short step to treating the dream itself as a symptom and to applying to dreams our method of interpretation that has been worked out for symptoms.
>
> This involves some psychological preparation of the patient. . . . He must adopt a completely impartial attitude to what occurs to him, since it is precisely this critical attitude which is responsible for his being unable, in the ordinary course of things, to achieve the desired unravelling of his dream or obsessional idea or whatever it may be. (pp. 100–101)

Decoding by free association was thus the method Freud pursued with neurotic symptoms and extended into the interpretation of dreams. No wonder, therefore, that this method has an especially strong emotional meaning for him, in comparison with a "holistic" method of interpretation. As he himself confessed, he arrived very late at a full realization of the importance of symbolism in dreams. In the first edition of *The Interpretation of Dreams,* his discussion was limited to a few pages and a single specimen dream. In 1914, Freud (who kept revising *The*

Interpretation of Dreams in successive editions) added an entirely new chapter on symbolism. In it he acknowledged his debt to his student, Stekel, and quoted extensively from Stekel's insights into dream symbolism. But his acknowledgment of Stekel's contribution was grudging. In 1925, for example, he wrote that Stekel had "perhaps damaged psychoanalysis as much as he benefitted it." Freud even went so far as to suspect that "every dreamer who has a grasp of symbols is a victim of schizophrenia" (p. 351). This is hardly an encouragement to a student of dreaming to make use of the dream's manifest content in gestalt or symbolic fashion!

Breaking down the dream into its elements, associating freely—that is, without reference to the dictates of judgment or conscience—was the method Freud had used in his own self-analysis. When it came to presenting dream interpretations, his own dreams were a "copious and convenient" source of illustrative material (p. 105). There was also another reason why he chose to present his own dreams and, in consequence, his own most intimate feelings, as the raw data for his treatise. Even though he had accumulated more than a thousand analyzed dreams from his patients, he felt that his own dreams were more suitable for exposition because they were obtained from "an approximately normal person, and relating to the multifarious occasions of daily life," instead of from neuropaths about whom a lengthy and often "highly bewildering" case history would be needed (p. 105).

This tradition of self-examination and introspection that Freud was using was a noble one, and, in fact, the main method of inquiry in psychology in Freud's time. Freud quotes a contemporary, Delboeuf, who wrote: "Every psychologist is under an obligation to confess even his own weaknesses, if he thinks it may throw light upon some obscure problem" (p. 105). Fechner, a prominent psychologist in Freud's day, had made excellent use of the introspectionist tradition to observe the gradations of sensory experience that accompany gradations in the physical stimulus, and to develop a formula that systematized the relationship between physical stimulus and physical response.

But Freud's presentation of his dreams and their associative connections was of an even more heroic kind than ever had been before, because he was offering to his readers his own mortifying and embarrassing experiences. Keeping strict account of one's own moral and professional failures is hard enough; presenting them as the raw material of a treatise on dreams must have been even harder. Nevertheless, Freud was mercilessly honest with himself and his readers. It was a part of the inquiry that Freud had started into the effect of our strong passions on our behavior. Even when a dream was clearly related to a painful, somatic stimulus, he kept at the analysis of it to show himself that it also expressed very painful feelings of humiliation vis-à-vis one of his colleagues. Perhaps the most touching example of Freud's honesty is his interpretation of the dream he had while suffering from very painful boils at the base of his scrotum. Freud dreamed that he was

> riding on a grey horse, timidly and awkwardly to begin with, as though I were only reclining. I met one of my colleagues, P., who was sitting high on a horse dressed in a tweed suit, and who drew my attention to something (probably my bad seat). I now began to find myself sitting more and more comfortably on my highly intelligent horse, and noticed that I was feeling quite at home up there.

Freud's wish not to have boils is expressed in his comfortable ride on the horse. But the dream also expressed the circumstance that his colleague, P., had been riding "the high horse" over Freud ever since he had taken over one of Freud's women patients. Freud was aware, incidentally, that some readers may have "doubts of the trustworthiness of 'self-analysis' of this kind; I shall be told that they leave the door open to arbitrary conclusions" (p. 105). Ironically, these words are prophetic: Freud's difficulty in accepting symbolic interpretations of manifest dream content and his bias in favor of the breakdown of dreams into associative elements is only one example of the "arbitrary rules" about manifest content that he imposed on dream interpretation.

Let us turn now to Freud's own sample dream, his dream about his patient, Irma. Presenting the dream text in full makes it possible for the reader to see if he or she can guess from the dream's manifest content what strangulated affect was bothering Freud, and to see if the reader's guess—made without reading Freud's own associative breakdown—corresponds with Freud's ultimate interpretation based on the dream's elements.

PREAMBLE

> During the summer of 1895 I had been giving psychoanalytic treatment to a young lady who was on very friendly terms with me and my family. It will be readily understood that a mixed relationship such as this may be a source of many disturbed feelings in a physician and particularly in a psychotherapist. While the physician's personal interest is greater, his authority is less; any failure would bring a threat to the old-established friendship with the patient's family. This treatment had ended in a partial success; the patient was relieved of her hysterical anxiety but did not lose all her somatic symptoms. At that time I was not yet quite clear in my mind as to the criteria indicating that a hysterical case history was finally closed, and I proposed a solution to the patient which she seemed unwilling to accept. While we were thus at variance, we had broken off the treatment for the summer vacation.— One day I had a visit from a junior colleague, one of my oldest friends, who

had been staying with my patient, Irma, and her family at their country resort. I asked him how he had found her and he answered: "She's better, but not quite well." I was conscious that my friend Otto's words, or the tone in which he spoke them, annoyed me. I fancied I detected a reproof in them, such as to the effect that I had promised the patient too much; and, whether rightly or wrongly, I attributed the supposed fact of Otto's siding against me to the influence of my patient's relatives, who, as it seemed to me, had never looked with favour on the treatment. However, my disagreeable impression was not clear to me and I gave no outward sign of it. The same evening I wrote out Irma's case history, with the idea of giving it to Dr. M. (a common friend who was at that time the leading figure in our circle) in order to justify myself. That night (or more probably the next morning) I had the following dream, which I noted down immediately after waking.

DREAM OF JULY 23RD–24TH, 1895

A large hall—numerous guests, whom we were receiving.—Among them was Irma. I at once took her on the side, as though to answer her letter and to reproach her for not having accepted my "solution" yet. I said to her: "If you still get pains, it's really only your fault." She replied: "If you only knew what pains I've got now in my throat and stomach and abdomen—it's choking me".—I was alarmed that after all I must be missing some organic trouble. I took her to the window and looked down her throat, and she showed signs of recalcitrance, like women with artificial dentures. I thought to myself that there was really no need for her to do that.—She then opened her mouth properly and on the right I found a big white patch; at another place I saw extensive whitish grey scabs upon some remarkable curly structures which were evidently modeled on the turbinal bones of the nose.—I at once called in Dr. M., and he repeated the examination and confirmed it. . . . Dr. M. looked quite different from usual; he was very pale, he walked with a limp and his chin was clean-shaven. . . . My friend Otto was now standing beside her as well, and my friend Leopold was percussing her through her bodice and saying: "She has a dull area low down on the left." He also indicated that a portion of the skin on the left shoulder was infiltrated. (I noticed this, just as he did, in spite of her dress.) . . . M. said: "There's no doubt it's an infection, but no matter; dysentery will supervene and the toxin will be eliminated." . . . We were directly aware, too, of the origin of the infection. Not long before, when she was feeling unwell, my friend Otto had given her an injection of a preparation of propyl, propyls . . . propionic acid . . . trimethylamin (and I saw before me the formula for this printed in heavy type). . . . Injections of that sort ought not to be made so thoughtlessly. . . . And probably the syringe had not been clean.

Freud tells us, incidentally, that this was the first of his dreams that he submitted to detailed interpretation. Amazingly (at least to this observer) he was convinced that the dream was uninterpretable without associations to each element. He writes:

No one who has read only the preamble and the content of the dream could have the slightest notion of what the dream meant. I myself had no notion. I was astonished at the symptoms of which Irma complained to me in the dream since they were not the same as those for which I had treated her. [A garden-variety obsessional defense which the very discoverer of defenses is surely using here!] I smiled at the senseless idea of an injection of propionic acid and at Dr. M.'s consoling reflections. Towards the end the dream seemed to me to be more obscure and compressed than it was at the beginning. In order to discover the meaning of all this it was necessary to undertake a detailed analysis. (p. 108)

But even without the daytime experiences that Freud presents in the preamble to his dream—his annoyance at his friend Otto's fancied reproof over Irma's being "not quite well" under Freud's psychoanalytic treatment—the central theme in the dream text is clear: Freud is not guilty of poor or ineffective treatment, but his friend Otto is. This message is inherent in the dream's manifest story without any further breakdown of elements. Irma is ill, Freud reproaches her for not "accepting his solution" to her illness; Freud is alarmed, calls in a consultant, and it turns out that Irma is ill because Otto had used some chemical (not psychonalaysis) and moreover had used a dirty syringe. Bad medical treatment, not psychoanalysis, is responsible for her illness.

Freud's own conclusion, after all his extensive associative connections to elements in the dream, is the same as its manifest message:

I was not responsible for the persistence of Irma's pains, but Otto was. Otto had in fact annoyed me by his remarks about Irma's incomplete cure, and the dream gave me my revenge by throwing the reproach back on him. The dream acquitted me of the responsibility for Irma's condition by showing that it was due to other factors—it produced a whole series of reasons. . . . *Thus its content was the fulfillment of a wish and its motive was a wish.* (Freud's italics) The whole plea—for the dream was nothing else—reminded one vividly of the defense put forward by the man who was charged by one of his neighbors with having given back a borrowed kettle in damaged condition. The defendant asserted first, that he had given it back undamaged; secondly, that the kettle had a hole in it when he borrowed it; and thirdly, that he had never borrowed a kettle at all from his neighbor. (pp. 118–120)

His Irma dream, then, was a product of a state of guilt, or, more accurately, a feeling of mortification at therapeutic failure, which Freud had at first warded off and then throttled during the preceding day. His "disagreeable impression" was not at all clear to him and he "gave no outward sign of it" (p. 106). The dream's content, however, amply avenges Freud on both his recalcitrant patient and his disapproving colleague. Why, then, did Freud need so elaborate a procedure as an element-by-element decoding to come to the dream's manifest central wish for revenge? It must be that his feeling of guilt or mortification, so apparent to us, was not really available to him. Indeed, as he describes his own experience, he turned away from his feelings and proceeded to write a lengthy account of Irma's case for Dr. M. Otto had "annoyed" him; but Freud's sense of justice rejected this annoyance as inappropriate to a "fancied reproach." The simplest phenomenological description of guilt indicated that it skirts a feeling of anger, but without the person being aware of more than a disagreeable impression, just as Freud reported. In any case, Freud was not clearly aware of *his* state of guilt until he had freely associated to the elements in the dream. Only then was the "meaning of the dream borne in upon" him (p. 118).

One wonders whether Freud's attachment to "free association" as opposed to holistic methods of dream analysis—and of grasping affects at work—did not become fixed as a result of his own patterns of affective management. In this connection, out of curiosity to see whether Freud's other dreams (which he analyzed in similar fashion) were also comprehensible from their manifest content, I made a list of dream themes. In 24 out of 31 dreams, the manifest theme was his career: his professional skill, as in Irma's case, or his hoped-for professorship and his envy of the colleagues who were thus acknowledged by their peers. It is easy to understand that the feelings of humiliated fury which are involved in the central theme of one's professional career are very difficult to experience fully—at least they are difficult for a "rational" man like Freud. The breakdown of each dream into its elements, associating freely to each of them, coming up only then with a compelling insight into one's own (morally unjustified) fury, could well have been the necessary procedure for Freud, although an emotionally uninvolved observer could get the point without such difficulty. At any rate, Freud was following his own experience when he built into his theoretical system the dictum that the manifest content of a dream cannot be the basis for its interpretation. And as we shall see, this dictum seriously hampered further dream research from 1900 to 1950 because it proclaimed in advance that any systematic study of manifest dreams was bound to be useless without associative breakdown as the means of correct interpretation.

In the chapters that follow his exposition of the Irma dream, Freud expounds the insights that have come to him with "the daylight of a sudden discovery."

> Dreams are not to be likened to the unregulated sounds that arise from a musical instrument struck by a blow of some external force instead of a player's hand; they are not meaningless, they are not absurd, they do not imply that one portion of our store of ideas is asleep while another portion is beginning to wake. On the contrary, they are psychical phenomena of complete validity—fulfillments of wishes; they can be inserted into the chain of intelligible waking mental acts; they are constructed by a highly complicated activity of the mind. (p. 122)

Freud devotes a chapter to the thesis that dreams are always wish fulfillments. In proof of this assertion he cites, first, dreams that are *undisguised* wish fulfillments. He points out that some dreams are convenience dreams, such as being in school (where one is expected) when one is oversleeping in the morning. In an amusing close to this chapter, Freud writes:

> I do not myself know what animals dream of. But a proverb, to which my attention was drawn by one of my students, does claim to know."what", asks the proverb, "do geese dream of?" And it replies:"Of maize." The whole theory that dreams are wish fulfillments is contained in these two phrases. (pp. 131–132)

But undisguised dreams are dreamed by children (and geese); or in the case of adults, they occur occasionally as convenience dreams. By implication, catching the emotional meaning of a dream without breaking it down into its elements is too simple a procedure to evoke much respect; instead, the complicated activities of the mind are needed to understand dreams. Once again, Freud's bias against emotions as compared to complicated ideational activities is apparent.

In order to defend his thesis that dreams are always wish fulfillments, Freud had to deal with two objections: that there are very unpleasant dreams, often frightening experiences, which can hardly express wishes; and that dreams are often so nonsensical and absurd, or about such emotionally indifferent matters, that they can hardly have to do with wishes. His answer to both of these objections is the same: The manifest dream may be anxious, but it *conceals* a wish; the manifest dream may appear to be about a triviality, but its breakdown will lead to a wish. By a process of circular reasoning, the breakdown system has become the *only* interpretive system to trust. Even if a dream looks as if it contains its wish in the manifest content, this is only a facade. Understandable dreams are like double agents in a spy story: never to be trusted!

Freud is at his most insightful in describing the way in which dream content represents the dreamer's affective life. He solves the conundrum implicit in the fact that dream content makes use of trivial or unnoticed parts of daytime experience but is actually about important emotional experiences—he solves that conundrum by showing that the trivial event in the dream is a distortion or disguise for the important one. A similar conundrum, that dreams make use of very recent daytime experiences but are also connected with earliest memories, is solved by the hypothesis that the recent event already must have some emotional significance, so that it resonates to similar childhood events. The recent event sets off a chain of memories leading to earliest throttled affects.

This observation becomes the basis from which Freud generalizes that *all* dreams are not only wish fulfillments but fulfillments of infantile wishes. These are the same infantile wishes that create neurotic symptoms.

In a monumental chapter on the "dream work," Freud deals with the process by which the latent dream thoughts are transformed into their manifest content. He expounds the translation system by which the latent dream thoughts are represented in a language of the dream. Freud's translation system depends heavily on the assumption that the dream work makes use of associative connections rather than "gestalt" apprehension of the meaning of the whole. His unit of observation, as we have seen before, is "ideas" rather than holistic affects. As a consequence, the translation process he describes first is "condensation." Having observed that the number of ideas that came to him from his dream was very much greater than the length of the dream itself—which is, as he says, "laconic" in comparison—Freud assumes that a process of condensation is at work by which many ideas are compressed into a single dream element. He is aware, of course, that this assumption is based on a postdreaming analysis, not on any direct observation of how dreams are actually formed. In using his method of free association to dream elements, Freud has thus confounded the observations made in the course of interpreting a dream with the process by which the dream is supposed to have evolved.

Another of the hypothetical dream-formation processes Freud described is the process of displacement, by means of which a trivial item gains incongruous "intensity," that is, large amounts of feeling. This is the mechanism by which dreams often have a distorted appearance. Still a third process of dream formation is one in which the logic of the dream's thoughts is expressed metaphorically. So, for instance, a causal connection is expressed by close proximity between two events; opposites are allowed to exist together without any contradiction; words are used as puns. A fourth method of transformation which he describes involves pictorial representation: Ideas are transformed into hallucinatory experiences or scenes that represent the dream's thoughts in images. These last two metaphorical and symbolic methods of transformation obviously do not depend on random associations between elements but on a holistic approach to the dream's interpretation.

The controversy over whether the dream's manifest content should be taken holistically, or whether it must always be regarded with suspicion, rests on whether condensation and displacement, or metaphorical and symbolic representation, are assumed as the processes that form the dream out of the dreamer's latent thoughts. In Volume 1 a similar question arose in connection with hysterical symptoms: Should they be understood symbolically, or are they formed by associative connections to otherwise unrelated ideas? Both processes of transformation could be seen to work in the case of hysterical symptoms. But in the case of dreams, Freud's dictum forbidding the interpretation of the manifest dream ignored two of the processes of dream formation that he himself had described.

This prejudice against symbolic transformation is most clearly apparent in Freud's treatment of the last of the processes constituting the dream work. This is the process of "secondary revision." Secondary revision comes into play when we are at the threshold between sleeping and waking. Freud observed that even when we are dreaming we often have the experience that "this is only a dream." Dreams also contain within their text a tendency to make the dream conform with the characteristics of waking thought. Thus some dreams occur that

> at a superficial view, may seem fantastically logical and reasonable; they start from a possible situation, carry it on through a chain of consistent modifications and—though far less frequently—bring it to a conclusion which causes no surprise. Dreams which are of such a kind have been subjected to a far-reaching revision by this psychical function [secondary revision] which is akin to waking thought. (p. 490)

Thus, even if a dream appears to be directly understandable because its affects are clear, that is a result of secondary revision masking latent meaning. Again, it is as though the process of dream formation behaves like a double agent in a spy story, always double-crossing the hero.

But perhaps the clearest expression of the neglect of affects in Freud's work (and subsequently in psychoanalysis) is observable in the fact that the section on affect amounts to only 27 pages in a book of 621 pages. Freud observes that the affects in dreams are the same as those in waking life. He further observes that although the ideational components of a dream have undergone displacement and condensation, *"the affects have remained unaltered"* (p. 460, Freud's italics). Freud observes, further, that many dreams are without affect. This fact he attributes to the struggle between opposing feelings within the person—these create a kind of emotional stalemate. Thus, even though, as we saw in his own Irma dream, the affects struggling with each other are clear and lively, their power is not considered theoretically.

STUDIES OF DREAM INTERPRETATION SINCE 1900

Among the most interesting studies are those that have attempted some experimental manipulation of the conditions under which dreams occur. For example, one of Freud's students, Herbert Silberer (1912/

1951), made a study of the dreams he had as he was on the threshold between waking and sleeping and forcing himself to maintain concentrated intellectual activity. He tells of making an accidental observation one day when he lay down after lunch and forced himself, against the pull of mounting drowsiness, to think of the difference between the views of Kant and Schopenhauer about time. In his drowsy state, he was surprised and somewhat frightened by the appearance of hallucinatory images of great vividness. Silberer called attention to the possibility that these hallucinatory images represented the dreamer's immediate state of discomfort resulting from his effort to stay awake and continue effective thinking. Silberer called these hallucinatory images "autosymbolic," in the sense that they referred to the dreamer's most immediate affective state. He called this "functional" symbolism, to distinguish it from the transformations of wishes which formed the "material" content of the dream. He demonstrated that the "labile balance" between sleeping and waking could itself be represented in symbolic perceptual scenes, as for example: "I was stepping across a brook with one foot, but drew it back again at once with the intention of remaining on this side" (p. 625).

Freud's treatment of Silberer's contribution is an illustration of how prejudiced he was against grasping directly the affects symbolized in dreams. He was particularly critical of the "abuses" (Freud's term, p. 505) to which Silberer's description of functional symbolism could be put. Once again, as with his treatment of Stekel, Freud dismissed Silberer's contribution with an ad hominem interpretation—as reflecting a "species of self-observation" which may be "particularly prominent in philosophical minds [with] delusions of observation" (p. 506). (The fact that Silberer committed suicide shortly after being read out of the Vienna Society contributed further to the subsequent neglect of his work. There is a most interesting "slip" on the part of the editors of the *Standard Edition* of Freud's work: Silberer's name is not indexed in Volume 5.) Freud's prejudice against grasping immediate affective states pushed him and psychoanalysis into the pursuit of the infantile wish by more intellectual means.

Freud's student, Federn (1952), also used his own experience of the transition between sleeping and waking to study dreaming. He observed how the altered state of the "body-ego" (a term Federn meant to refer to the self) creates transient alterations of experience resembling depersonalization and estrangement. Federn went on to hypothesize that intense feeling states could also alter the relation of experience to the self and thereby create very frightening experiences, as if one were crazy.

Kubie and Margolin (1942) picked up the implication in these observations by Silberer and Federn that borderline states of consciousness themselves might be states in which affects are more accessible than they are in waking life. Kubie and Margolin devised a special technique for inducing hypnagogic reveries in their patients: They used the rhythm of the patient's breathing sounds as a monotonous fixating stimulus to induce partial sleep. They found that their procedure did "loosen" the patients and so might be used as an adjunct to psychoanalysis, in which Kubie and Margolin had both been trained.

Kubie (1943) reported a case in which a patient of his was greatly helped in 17 sessions, of which five were long hypnagogic reveries induced by this method. The patient had previously had a year and a half of ordinary psychoanalytic treatment, but was now in acute distress. Kubie reported that the free association process was much facilitated by the induced reverie state, and the patient was able to capture memories and feelings that previously had been inaccessible. These findings take us straight back to Breuer and Freud's early observations about the role of hypnoid states in the formation of symptoms. But principally because Freud had abandoned the notion of hypnoid state as a factor in neurosis (and had fused the theory of symptom formation with the theory of cure), adjunctive methods of treatment that included hypnoid states were looked on with suspicion by classical psychoanalysis. They were too close to the use of hypnosis as a therapy, which Freud had found inferior to the more "radical" talking-out use of hypnosis. It is only in relatively recent times that common ground is once again being sought between psychoanalysis and therapies that make use of hypnoid states (Brenman & Gill, 1947).

Some of Freud's early students, in fact, used hypnosis as a means of studying dream content (Rapaport, 1951). One kind of experimental procedure placed the person under hypnosis and suggested that he or she would later dream of some sexual experience—such as, for instance, having some form of forbidden sex. The experimenter also suggested that the person forget his suggestion. (The rationale for this procedure was that it paralleled Freud's idea that we dream of neglected or repressed ideas.) The expectation was that the dreams would contain symbolic transformations of the suggested sexual content. So, for instance, in a famous instance cited by Freud, Schroetter (1951) suggested to a young woman (E.) that she dream of homosexual intercourse with her friend (L.). E. then dreamed that L. appeared in a "dirty cafe," holding a threadbare suitcase with a sticker on it that read "For ladies only." The symbolic representation of woman's vagina by a suitcase and the symbol dirty cafe for forbidden oral intercourse are easily identifiable.

With regard to this experimental procedure, however, the question arose whether dreams induced in this way are really the same as those occurring naturally. In fact, one would expect that dreams that occur when a person is under hypnotic influence would have a special character of their own. In recent years it has been demonstrated, by the simple technique of asking people, that their hypnotic dreams and their ordinary dreams are quite different experiences. As we shall see in Chapter 3, the interpersonal involvement in hypnosis is itself a powerful source of affect and is dramatically transformed in dreams. The symbols are, as always, perfectly clear to an observer, although not to the dreamer.

Ironically, in view of Freud's prejudice against the dream work of symbolic transformation, it is the study of dream symbolism that has had the greatest impetus since Freud's time as well as the greatest influence on our culture. One important study, for example, actually spelled out the similarities between dreams and poetry. Ella Freeman Sharpe (1949), a nonmedical psychoanalyst who came into the psychoanalytic movement from the study of literature, called attention to the fundamental similarity between the workings of dream symbolism and the laws of poetic diction. (Sharpe, it should be noted in passing, simply used the dream's manifest content regardless of Freud's rules.) She reminds us, with a quotation from Milton, that poetic diction should be "simple, sensuous and passionate." This is because, Sharpe says, "the poet's task is to communicate *experience*" (p. 19, Sharpe's italics). "To this end," Sharpe continues,

> poetic diction prefers picturesque imagery to the enumeration of facts, it avoids the generic term and selects the particular. It is averse to lengthiness and dispenses with conjunction and relative pronoun where possible. It substitutes epithets for phrases. By means such as these a poem appeals to the ear and eye and becomes an animated canvas. (p. 19)

Sharpe then shows us how the poetic devices of simile, metaphor, metonymy, synecdoche, and onomatopoeia are used in dreams. She illustrates the use of simile and metaphor in a dream that the dreamer had while mourning the loss of a beloved person. The dream used music to restore lost love, as Shakespeare understood when he wrote: "If music be the food of love, play on." Here is its text (I have indicated simile and metaphor in brackets):

> I was at a concert and yet the concert was like a feeding [simile]. I could see the music pass before my eyes like pictures [simile]. The music pictures passed like ships in the night [simile]. There were two sorts of pictures, white mountains with softly rounded tops [metaphor for breast], and others following them were tall and pointed [metaphor for penis].

Sharpe interprets the ships that pass in the night as metaphors for the "great parents . . . friendly to each other" but no longer available to comfort the dreamer.

Sharpe illustrates the devices of metaphor in dreams. In metonymy a name that has a usual connection with a thing is used for the thing itself—as, for example, the bench or bar for the profession of law. So a "slatey-colored" face in a dream was a reference to death via tombstones which are made of slate. Synecdoche, in which a part of the object does duty for the whole, is illustrated by a dream in which "scarlet pimpernel" represents the breast; and onomatopoeia, in which the sound of a word echoes its sense, is illustrated by a dream in which "Iona cathedral" meant "I own a cathedral," and by a dream in which "sandwich" meant the "sand" (on the beach) and "which" meant a "witch." Sharpe summarizes her brilliant review of the similarities between poetry and dreaming by reminding us that the "basis of language is implied metaphor and that we all learned our mother tongue phonetically" (p. 39). In this approach, moreover, she is clearly basing her work on the social nature of humanity rather than on the systems of "excitation."

Three other important lines of Freudian investigation into dreaming can be discerned since 1900. These are: first, the analysis of manifest dream content from normal persons; second, the analysis of the manifest dream content of disturbed people; and finally, cross-cultural studies of dreams. All three lines of inquiry have yielded findings that Freud might well have predicted, had he not effectively barred speculation about manifest dreams.

Calvin Hall (Hall & VandeCastle, 1966) has been the person most responsible for the description of dreaming by normal people in the United States. By now Hall has collected more than 10,000 dream reports by simply asking people to record their dreams in the morning. Hall has analyzed the texts for a variety of simple, basic questions, such as the difference between men and women in the gender of the characters they dream about and in dream content. Hall and Domhoff (1964), for example, having looked at the results of 11 previous studies, found a "ubiquitous sex difference" in the dreams of 1,399 men and 1,418 women. Men dream about men; women's dreams are inhabited equally by characters of both sexes. (Similar findings have been observed in the dreams of the Hopi in our Southwest and Yiv Yaront in Australia.) Moreover, Hall and Domhoff found that aggression in the dreams of men was most often directed toward other males, whereas the aggression in the dreams of women was equally divided as to the sex of its target. Hall interprets men's greater aggressiveness toward other men as a consequence of the Oedipus complex, in which another male is the principal rival. He finds, in support of this notion, that men's dreams are more often about male "strangers" than women's; women dream more often of familiar people and more often (than men) of family members. Women's dreams are friendlier than men's.

One normative study of dreams in a midwestern American city (Kramer, Whitman, & Winget, 1970) is particularly instructive because it made use of a psychoanalytic method of scoring verbal material for the affect implied in the content (Gottschalk & Gleser, 1969), as well as the Hall-VandeCastle scoring method. Striking differences were found between men and women. Men had more dreams scorable for covert hostility directed outward, for aggression, success, misfortunes occurring to them, castration anxiety, outdoor scenes, and work references. Each of these variables clearly reflects men's role in society. Women reported more dreams than men; they also reported more dreams with people in them and more people per dream. Women had more dreams scorable for friendly acts, misfortunes occurring to others, emotions, indoor scenes, and family references. T. Parson's (1964) "instrumental" and "expressive" personality dimensions, Bakan's (1966) "agency" and "communion" societal roles, are thus clearly descriptive not only of the social behavior of men and women but of their dreams. These findings are clearly assimilable to Freud's notion that the Oedipus complex is more central for men than for women.

In still another study, Hall and VandeCastle examined the manifest dreams of college students, guided by the Freudian notion that men's dreams should have more reference to castration anxiety, whereas women's dreams should be more concerned with penis envy. Clear-cut criteria for the existence of castration anxiety were established on which independent judges could agree. These included themes of actual or threatened loss or defect of the dreamer's body, or inability to use his penis. The criteria for penis envy included acquisition within the dream of phallic objects; and admiration or envy of phallic objects. As predicted, men's dreams had more references to castration anxiety than women's; conversely, women's dreams had more references to penis envy than men's. Another analysis of these data is quite cogent: 50% of the women had no references to castration anxiety in their dreams; this was true of only 8% of the men.

Studies of the manifest dreams of neurotic and psychotic patients also yield results that are in keeping with Freudian predictions. As one example of this kind of study, Beck (1967), who has more recently developed cognitive approaches to depression, observed that the dreams of depressed patients (who are more often women than men) were full of references to masochistic content. He developed a scale for assessing dreams along this dimension. A dream is scored as having masochistic content if the dreamer has a negative representation of the self, for example, "I was a bum"; if the dream is about physical discomfort or injury; about being thwarted, deprived, physically attacked, verbally attacked; being excluded, superseded, or abandoned; being lost; being punished; or about failure. Dreams of depressed patients, scored by judges who did not know the patients' diagnoses, more often contained masochistic content than dreams of other kinds of patients. Interestingly enough, depressed patients continued to have dreams with masochistic content even after they had clinically improved.

Another study (Langs, 1966) compared the manifest content of three groups of women psychiatric patients: hystericals, paranoid schizophrenics, and depressed patients. Again the dreams were assessed by judges who did not know the patients' diagnoses. Hystericals' dreams are occupied with themes of bodily injury, with open sexuality, and with interaction between the dreamer and other people. Paranoid schizophrenic dreams are full of fighting and of a view of the environment as traumatic or overwhelming; there were fewer interactions with others. Psychotic depressive dreams were relatively brief and barren compared to the other two categories, but they centered on family members: "I dreamed I was with my family as it was in former times."

In still another kind of study of patients' dreams (Lewis, 1959), I compared two women patients who differ very much in their cognitive style. Patient Z. has a field-independent cognitive style. Her judgments are relatively uninfluenced by the prevailing framework; she has a self that is organized so that it is the reference point for her experience; in everyday personality description she would be called "self-centered." Patient A., in contrast, has a field-dependent way of perceiving herself in relation to the world. She is much influenced by the prevailing framework, and she has a self that is heavily involved in relations with others. Patient A.'s symptoms are of depression with hysteria; Patient Z.'s diagnosis is more in the paranoid schizoid direction. Each patient's dreams clearly reflected her cognitive style—that is, the characteristic organization of the self in relation to the world. So, for instance, Z. had many dreams in which she saw herself or had a "bird's-eye view" of herself as if she were an observer of the scene. Along with this frequent self-imaging, there was a shaky sense of identity in Z.'s dreams. So, for example, she dreamed that a character was talking, but his "talking was in my head and didn't come out of his mouth." A., in contrast, had dreams in which the protagonist was taken for granted to be herself, in her own form, not needing further description. A.'s dreams were full of kinesthetic-visceral experience, in contrast to Z.'s, in which there was much distancing of the self from experience. A.'s dreams were more mundane or "homier"; Z.'s more bizarre, in keeping also with their personal styles of existence, as well as with their psychiatric symptoms.

Cross-cultural studies of dreaming also confirm what is implicit in

Freud's description of dreaming—that dreams are about universal emotional conflicts. Freud collaborated in an early study of dreams in folklore (Freud & Oppenheim, 1911).[1] In this paper, many instances are cited in which folk wisdom in effect interprets a dream psychoanalytically. Here is an amusing example from South Slav folk tradition:

> A girl got up from her bed and told her mother that she had a most strange dream. "Well, what did you dream, then?" asked the mother.
> "How shall I tell you? I don't know myself what it was—some sort of long and red and blunted thing."
> "Long means a road," said her mother reflectively, "a long road; red means joy; but I don't know what blunted can mean."
> The girl's father, who was getting dressed meanwhile, and was listening to everything that the mother and daughter were saying, muttered at this, more or less to himself, "It sounds rather like my cock." (pp. 180–181)

As one example of a sophisticated cross-cultural study of dreams, let us look at a study by Roy D'Andrade (1961). D'Andrade was impressed by the frequent ethnographical accounts of the way in which dreams comforted people who felt isolated and unloved. There are ethnographers' accounts, moreover, of primitive peoples who use dreams psychotherapeutically. So, for instance, D'Andrade quotes Wallace (1958, pp. 237–238), who observed that the Iroquois were psychologically sophisticated. They recognized that there were

> conscious and unconscious parts of the mind. They knew the great force of unconscious desires, and were aware that the frustration of these desires could cause mental and physical (psychosomatic) illness . . . and that the best method of relief was to give the frustrated idea satisfaction, either directly or symbolically.

D'Andrade therefore formulated the hypothesis that where the culture is preoccupied with dreams that control supernatural powers, there should also be indications of cultural pressure on the individual to be independent and self-sufficient. D'Andrade found that cultures in which the son moves a greater distance away from his parental group on marriage were also those in which dreams are used to control supernatural powers. Similarly, the mode of subsistence economy is related to the use of dreams to control superior force. Hunting and fishing econo-

---

[1]Oppenheim died in Theresienstadt. His wife survived and had somehow managed to preserve the manuscript of this joint paper. The Oppenheims' daughter brought it forward after her mother's death in 1956. The Holocaust is thus indirectly responsible for the long delay in the publication of this paper, which Freud had promised in a footnote to the third edition (1911) of *The Interpretation of Dreams*. Freud apparently abandoned the project after Oppenheim had joined Adler in resigning from the Vienna Psychoanalytic Society in 1911.

mies stress individual self-reliance and independence much more than agricultural economies, which put more stress on obedience to group laws. This difference is built into the differing requirements for survival: Crops must be reliably (obediently) tended; hunting large game animals, in contrast, requires initiative and self-reliance rather than obedience. By the same token hunting and fishing economies place much stress upon the individual, whereas agricultural economies allow more group sharing of stress. Eighty percent of hunting and fishing societies use dreams to control supernatural powers; only 20% of agricultural economies use dreams in this way!

It will be remembered that my patient Z., a field-independent perceiver, had dreams in which she was (wishfully) in control of events, in contrast to the more passive role of my field-dependent patient, A. There is also evidence (Witkin & Berry, 1975) that people in hunting and fishing economies are, on the average, more field-independent perceivers than people in agricultural economies. D'Andrade's finding about the difference in their dreams also fits their differing cognitive styles.

It is a measure of Freud's genius that the observations he made on his dreams can thus be confirmed in worldwide cross-cultural studies. The theoretical structure that Freud built around his observations was avowedly tentative, although he did not really use it in that spirit. As we shall see in the next chapter, the discovery of REM periods has rendered Freud's theoretical system practically useless. But it has not invalidated his observations, which, along with the new information about dreaming, still challenge us to develop a comprehensive theory of people's emotions.

CHAPTER 2

The Discovery of the REMS
The Problem of Freud's Theory

Freud's insights about the emotional meaning of dream content (like his clinical observations about hysterical symptoms) were placed by him in a theoretical straitjacket that not only created a schism among his followers but also discouraged fresh observations about dreams. The blow to Freud's theory of dreams that resulted from the discovery of the REMS was felt as a relief by some clinicians, including myself, who had long been irritated by classical psychoanalysis's slavish adherence to "rules" forbidding dream interpretation outside the analytic situation. The discovery of the REMS has actually made it possible to study dreaming on the spot, with control over presleep emotional input. As we shall see in the next chapter, a firsthand study (in which I was one of a team of researchers) of REM period dreams collected from normal people demonstrates the freshness and vitality of Freudian dream interpretation, although dream theory remains obscure.

In this chapter we shall look first at Freud's theory of dreams as he propounded it in Chapter 7 of *The Interpretation of Dreams.* A close look at Freud's theorizing is necessary because it illustrates the difficulties of bringing dream interpretation and neurotic symptoms into a common theoretical system without focusing on the power of emotional ties. We shall see how experimental attempts to confirm Freud's theory failed even before the discovery of the REMS, and we shall look in detail at the way in which the discovery of the REMS finally disconfirmed Freud's theory.

CHAPTER 7 OF *The Interpretation of Dreams*

Chapter 7 has become the would-be psychoanalyst's introduction to and groundwork of psychoanalytic theory. In this chapter Freud sets out not only a theory of dreaming but a theory of neurotic symptom formation as well. It is from this chapter that the rigidities of Freudian thinking have grown, even though Freud explicitly described his theory as tentative.

Freud's theory of dreams, like his theory of neurotic symptoms, is based on the model of the reflex arc, S–R: A stimulus (S) enters over sensory pathways and requires to be discharged over motor pathways in the form of a response (R). Discharge is in "movement" or in "expression of emotion." (Here Freud is making reference to Darwin's idea of emotions as adaptive residuals.) The evoked S resulting from a need requires an "experience of satisfaction" as its R. If satisfaction is obtained, then the next time the need arises it

> will seek to re-cathect the mnemic [memory] image of the perception . . . to re-establish the situation of the original satisfaction. An impulse of this kind is what we call a wish; the reappearance of the perception is the fulfillment of the wish. . . . there was [thus] a primitive state of the apparatus in which wishing ended in hallucinating. (p. 566)

This mode of discharge, primitive and regressive, is Freud's notion of how infants respond. As we shall see in later chapters, it was the version of infancy current in Freud's time—the same set of ideas that moved William James to speak of infant experience as one of "buzzing, blooming confusion." We now know that infants are by no means so "primitively" organized as Freud had supposed. It is also clear from this quotation that Freud regarded "wishing" as something like a raw physiological instinct. This is a solipsist view of humanity: People are governed from infancy by the instinct to receive their own gratifications. But our current knowledge of the social nature of infants makes it more useful to consider wishing as an early social-emotional response.

From the very earliest moments, however, our gratifications (emotions) are also blocked. An infant wants the breast; discharge of this impulse is delayed; the infant then hallucinates. The infant, of course, can also do something more efficient, about which Freud has very little to say other than that the infant develops "thinking" or "reality testing." He (she) learns, as a result of deprivations, to develop a "reality principle." This reality principle Freud also calls a "secondary system," to contrast it with the "primary-process" pleasure-principle system he has hypothesized for the infant's first responses. Here Freud is very clear about the superiority of thinking over emotions (wishing), at the same time that he writes: "All this activity of thought merely constitutes a roundabout path to wish-fulfillment which has been made necessary by [frustrating] experience" (p. 567). The two psychical systems that thus emerge are the "primary-process" and the "secondary" systems; the former is organized to seek discharge, the latter to inhibit the discharge of energy. The secondary system is clearly superior to the primary.

> Dreams which fulfill their wishes along the short path of regression have merely preserved for us in that respect a sample of the psychical apparatus' primary method of working, a method which is abandoned as being inefficient. What once dominated waking life, while the mind was young and incompetent, seems now to have been banished into the night. (p. 567)

Freud is quite explicit about the tentativeness of these formulations.

> The mechanics of these processes are quite unknown to me; anyone who wished to take these ideas seriously would have to look for physical analogies to them and find a means of picturing the movements that accompany excitation of neurons. (p. 599)

Each of us, Freud theorizes, has a storehouse of hallucinatory experiences resulting from the blockage of the pleasure principle. These experiences, expecially since they occurred preverbally, have no words to express them; they remain forever inaccessible in what Freud calls "primary repression."

> In consequence of the belated appearance of the secondary process, the core of our being, consisting of unconscious wishful impulses, remains inaccessible to the understanding and inhibition of the preconscious; the part played by the latter is restricted once and for all to directing along the most expedient paths the wishful impulses that arise from the unconscious. (p. 603)

How, then, does a dream actually form, once we are adults? What happens is this: During the daytime "we come upon an idea that will not bear criticism; we break off: we drop the cathexis of attention" (p. 593). Such a train of thought is then "preconscious"; but it may connect itself with that storehouse of primary repressions. The ideas from which we turned away are "drawn into the unconscious" by an "attraction" to "primary repressions" already existing. In addition to this attraction, thoughts are kept operating in "primary process" because the dreamer has a wish (or need) that keeps the dream thoughts closer to their "unconscious connection." Dream content is thus indirectly governed by the state of sleep: Dreams are formed in order to prevent awakening; they are thus the "guardians of sleep." The preconscious thoughts, as a result of their unconscious connection, are expressed in a dream that forms according to "primary-process" wish-fulfillment laws of thinking, including hallucinatory experiences of the wished-for gratifications.

When the preconscious thought meets the unconscious storehouse, the "train of thought undergoes a series of transformations which we can no longer recognize as normal psychical processes and which leads to a result that bewilders us—a psychopathological structure" (p. 595).

At this point Freud again lists the varieties of dream work. Significantly, in this final listing, symbolic transformations play no part at all. Freud emphasizes, rather, the work of condensation and displacement. He insists, in fact, that facilitating "regression to images" is *not* the main point of dream work (p. 597). It is interesting to observe, in this connection, that Ernest Jones's (1910/1950) résumé of Freud's work on dreams explicitly cites condensation and displacement (distortion) as the two major forms of dream work.

Freud had undertaken his study of dreams to throw light on hysteria and other neurotic formations. Actually, in propounding his theory of dreams, he used the insights gained from his study of hysteria to solve the problem of why "primary-process" thinking occurs in dreams. His analysis of the process of dreaming and of the process of hysterical symptom-formation uncovered similar mechanisms:

> Normal thoughts have been submitted to abnormal treatment: *they have been transformed into the symptoms by means of condensation and the formation of compromises, by way of superficial associations and in disregard of contradictions, and, also, it may be, along the path of regression* (Freud's italics). In view of the complete identity between the characteristic features of the dream-work and those of physical activity which issues in psychoneurotic symptoms, we feel justified in carrying over to dreams the conclusions we have been led to by hysteria.
>
> We accordingly borrow the following thesis from the theory of hysteria: A normal train of thought is only submitted to abnormal psychical treatment of the sort we have been describing if an unconscious wish, derived from infancy and in a state of repression, has been transferred on to it. (p. 598)

As Freud immediately points out, however, the assumption that the motive power for a dream invariably originates from the unconscious "cannot be proved to hold generally, though neither can it be disproved" (pp. 597–598).

From the theory of psychoneuroses Freud also derived the fact that "only sexual wishful impulses from infancy, which have undergone repression . . . are able to furnish the motive force for the formation of neurotic symptoms of every kind" (pp. 605–606). But he leaves it

> an open question whether these sexual and infantile factors are equally required in the theory of dreams: I will leave that theory incomplete at this point, since I have already gone beyond what can be demonstrated in assuming that dream wishes are invariably derived from the unconscious. (p. 606)

What Freud does derive, finally, from his study of dreams and the connection he has made between dreams and hysterical symptoms is that *"what is suppressed continues to exist in normal people as well as abnormal, and remains capable of psychical functioning"* (p. 608, Freud's italics). There follows then a very famous quotation: "The interpretation of dreams is the royal road to a knowledge of the unconscious activities of the mind" (p. 608). In Freud's theorizing, dreams have become the royal road to these unconscious activities rather than to feelings that "the moral side of [our] nature" (p. 478) found acceptable.

How inadequate Freud's theoretical structure was to support the tremendous wealth of his observations is perhaps most apparent in two of the phenomena with which he had considerable difficulty in *The Interpretation of Dreams*. The first of these was the phenomenon of punishment or anxiety dreams. The second was the proposition that all dreams are formed out of infantile wishes remaining inaccessible in the memory storehouse. (In the case of this second principle, he was aware, as noted above, that he had already gone beyond the demonstrable.)

In the matter of punishment dreams, Freud changed his mind in later revisions of his book on dreams, and came to believe that there is a punishment wish—or as he called it, still later, "primary masochism." This is a derivative of our "death instinct," which, in turn, rests upon the tendency of all living matter to discharge excitations into quiescence. In a theoretical system based on discharge of excitations, the mechanism of punishment wishes remains the work of discharge, but now there are two discharge systems—gratifications based on death and on life instincts.

If Freud's theoretical system is held in abeyance for the moment, and punishment wishes examined simply as a phenomenon of feelings, then it becomes clear that they are what one experiences in a state of guilt. One's transgressions appear to demand that one expiate or discharge one's guilt by appropriate punishment. Looking only a little more deeply into this experience, it is easy to see that punishment wishes often maintain our emotional ties to the people we love. Punishment simultaneously discharges an obligation to them and to ourselves. Once we have expiated or been punished then we are once again lovable, no longer culpable. But a theoretical system based on the activity of neurons has great difficulty in accounting for behavior such as this, which is based on emotional ties.

In addition to its narrow technical base, Freud's theory suffers from his prejudice against holistic feeling–cognition states and his predilection for the breakdown of elements or ideas so as to retrieve the "unconscious" ideation. It is thus no wonder that the psychoanalytic enterprise becomes an intellectual task of great magnitude. Simple catharsis of feelings pales into insignificance by comparison.

The second difficulty Freud encountered in his theoretical system had to do with his insistence that dreams are formed only out of infantile wishes. Freud had proposed, moreover, in his *Three Essays on Sexuality,* that the gratification of our earliest infantile wishes also evokes the sexual wishes; in fact, he insisted that he had never said so, although this is obviously what he had implied: The forbidden, sexual, infantile instinct is what dreams so tortuously disguise. But if, as I have suggested, the notion that our earliest needs are sexual is transformed to mean that our earliest needs are social, then the concept of infantile sexuality sheds some of the difficulties that have surrounded it. Dream content, like neurotic symptoms, can be understood as evoked by guilt and shame, and these affective states, in turn, are ways in which we attempt to restore lost emotional ties. In this view, the psychoanalytic enterprise need not (although it may) focus on the reconstruction of the past (infantile sexuality), but it may also operate effectively by analyzing the present emotional dilemma.

The theoretical system Freud built as the result of his study of dreams was an elegant one that included the instigation, content, and forgetting of dreams in a single explanatory model: a conflict between two systems. This theoretical model, although it was meant to be discarded when new information became available, actually became a straitjacket. A set of rules evolved for understanding dreams which were as follows: (1) Manifest dreams are not interpretable; (2) a dream is not fully interpreted until one has unearthed the infantile sexual wish that evoked the dream; and (3) dreams are forgotten only as a result of repression. The implications of this set of rules for psychoanalysis as a form of therapy were equally constricting, especially since dream interpretation became an integral part of the reconstruction of "primary repressions."

Just how dogmatic dream interpretation has become in psychoanalytic practice is exemplified in the way Freud treated Dora's first important dream during their work together. Dora (see Volume 1, Chapter 3) had been in a state of "mortification" (Freud's term) over being betrayed by the persons she had loved best in the world—her father, Frau K., and Herr K. Dora dreamed that her father, faced with a conflict of loyalty, had chosen to side with and protect his children. This is what Dora had been demanding of him, although uncertain herself whether she was justified. But Freud was set upon finding the infantile wish. By breaking up the manifest content of the dream into its elements, Freud came upon Dora's early masturbation and, underneath her unrequited love of Herr K., her incestuous love for her father. Dora responded to Freud's line of dream interpretation by abruptly leaving treatment.

In this case account Freud is particularly defensive about his method of dream interpretation. He "interrupts" the account to say that his

> theory would have been more certain of general acceptance if I had contented myself with maintaining that every dream had a meaning [and] then gone on to say that the meaning of a dream turned out to be of as many different sorts as the processes of waking thought; that in one case it would be a fulfilled wish, in another a realized fear, or again a reflection persisting on into sleep, or an intention [as in the instance of Dora's dream] or a piece of creative thought during sleep, and so on. (pp. 67–68)

One wishes indeed that Freud had maintained this degree of flexibility. To have demonstrated that dreams express our conflicts was surely enough of a contribution without an elaborate (and ultimately useless) theoretical structure.

Progress in understanding dreams since Freud's time has come mainly out of disregard for Freud's theoretical system, and out of a sensitive appreciation for the affective modes of experience that dreams represent. Direct tests of Freudian theory have not had much success; in contrast, Freud's observations about dream content have been widely confirmed.

One of the most widely quoted "tests" of Freudian dream theory is the Poetzl phenomenon (Poetzl, Allers, & Teller, 1960). Poetzl presented pictures of everyday scenes to people tachistoscopically—that is, for intervals too brief for the person to be able to grasp the whole picture. Poetzl then asked his subjects to draw what they had seen in the picture. He then examined their subsequent dreams with the prediction, which he confirmed, that the unnoticed details of the picture would be represented in the dream content, whereas the details that had been noticed would be absent. The controversy that developed over the Poetzl phenomenon illustrates how easy it has been for Freud's original observations on affects to become blurred. Poetzl himself understood his findings on a physiological level. He postulated that there is a fundamental equivelance between brain damage and the impoverished perception resulting from too brief exposure to a stimulus; he theorized that these unperceived parts of experience are nevertheless "registered" in the physiological system. Dreams then develop these unperceived but registered experiences after the analogy of an underexposed photographic film that is later developed in a darkroom. Poetzl formulated a "law of exclusion": Consciously perceived experiences are excluded from dream content; dreams deal only with unperceived experience.

As one can see, there is no more than a faint parallel between Freud's ideas and Poetzl's. (It should be noted that Freud was unimpressed by the supposed parallel between his thinking and that of Poetzl.) The emotionally indifferent or unnoticed perceptions that Freud identified as suitable covers for an emotional experience are like Poetzl's "registered" unperceived elements only in being unperceived. Freud's concept of repression as central to dream formation is not at all like Poetzl's idea that dreaming permits some restoration of originally brain-damaged perception. From the fact that emotional conflict can make some experiences unnoticed it does not follow that all unnoticed experiences are connected to emotional conflict. Nevertheless, because Poetzl had observed that unconscious stimuli are operative in dreaming, and without regard to the fact that Poetzl's "unconscious" had nothing to do with Freud's, the repetition of Poetzl's experiment under better-controlled conditions was undertaken as research into psychoanalytic dream theory (C. Fisher, 1956). Part of what seemed so attractive was the possibility of quantifying "preconscious perception"—that is, perception without awareness—even though the emotional basis for the preconscious perception was not examined.

Shevrin and Luborsky (1958) performed a replication of Poetzl's experiment under very carefully controlled conditions. One of their purposes was to construct a "reliable measure of preconscious perception" (p. 286). They showed a slide of a scene in ancient Rome at an exposure of $1/50$ second. They then obtained on-the-spot drawings and a verbal description of what their 27 subjects recalled of the briefly exposed picture. Subjects were asked to write down their subsequent dreams; those subjects who did not recall any dreams were invited to close their eyes and tell about what "pictures"—came to mind. (These pictures or images were analyzed in the same way as the reported dreams.)

What Shevrin and Luborsky found, however, was contrary to the predictions from Poetzl's "law" of exclusion: The number of elements consciously grasped during the tachistoscopic exposure had no relation to the number of elements reported in the dreams, and the particular elements consciously grasped were *more* likely to appear in dreams than the elements not recalled. Faced with this failure to replicate Poetzl's findings, Shevrin and Luborsky undertook other statistical treatments of their data that reflected a modified version of Poetzl's hypothesis. But a later replication attempt also failed. No one has found an explanation for the discrepancy between these results and Poetzl's observations. The finding that perceived stimuli find their way into dreams is itself no surprise, nor does it go contrary to Freudian dream theory, which does not require that all dream stimuli be unperceived.

In any case, one result of the much studied Poetzl phenomenon and of the contradictory findings about it was that not only Freudian theory but Freud's observations were thrown into doubt. Once again, the affective phenomena he described tended to be overlooked as a consequence of theorizing about the "unconscious" as if it were only an intellectual function.

FREUD'S THEORY AND THE DISCOVERY OF THE REMS

Let us begin with a brief sketch of essential information about the REM period.[1] We now know that all mammals, including ourselves, spend a good portion of their lives in a cyclically recurring physiological state that is neither ordinary sleeping nor waking, a "third state" in which human beings dream. Dreaming is thus a concomitant of a biological function "given" to all mammals. This third state is sometimes called "rapid eye movement state" because the eyes are moving as if they were viewing some action, or "paradoxical sleep" because it is a state in which there is both arousal and shutdown of physiological functions, or "D-state" because when people are aroused from it they most often say that they have been dreaming. In fact, the direction of eye movement—up, down, right, left—has been observed to match the content of the dream scenes reported by the dreamer, and the intensity of the eye movement activity has been matched to the busyness of the dream's content.

These bursts of rapid eye movements were discovered accidentally in the course of monitoring the physiology of sleep. The sensitive electronic recording devices that had become available in the first decades of the twentieth century were being used to monitor the electroencephalography of sleep. It had already been established that normal sleep varies progressively in "depth" during the night. Deep sleep early in the night gives way to lighter and lighter sleep toward morning, and this progression is signaled by different patterns on the electroencephalogram labeled Stage 4 (delta) for deep sleep, through Stages 3 and 2 for lighter sleep, into Stage 1 (alpha) which is the lightest sleep—not too dissimilar from waking drowsiness. REM periods occur during Stage 1 or "light sleep," although, paradoxically, people may be harder to awaken in Stage 1 than in deeper stages if awakening is attempted during a REM period in which they are deeply absorbed in a dream experience.

The REMS is also paradoxical in being a period of simultaneous

---

[1]A more detailed, authoritative summary may be found in Snyder (1967).

physiological activation and shutdown. The state regularly involves erections of the penis; respiration is irregular and more rapid, brain temperature is increased. Simultaneously, there is a shutdown of gross muscular activity—for example, there is a loss of muscle tonus in the neck and chin.

Some variety of electrical stimulation is being fed from the brainstem into the visual cortex during the REMS. The chemical trigger for this electrical stimulation is unknown, but it is now hypothesized that some neurohumoral substance builds up in the nervous system which the REMS regularly discharges (Dement, 1969). Being deprived of REM periods, for example, makes the nervous system more irritable or excitable—more likely to go into convulsions. The REMS is thus a recurring "discharge" time that is somehow—although no one knows how—useful to the mamalian organism.

Let us now look at how the discovery of the REMS speaks against Freud's theory of dreaming. That theory postulated that a dream is instigated by some repression-connected experience seeking a second chance for expression during sleep. The discovery that people dream regardless of their immediately preceding emotional state is a direct blow to this theory.

If REM periods were instigated by the day's residue of emotional conflict, the number of REM periods or the time spent in REM sleep should be related to the degree of emotional arousal during the preceding day. Instead, the number of REM periods each night is relatively stable—there are, on the average, four REM periods in each night's sleep. If anything, the night after emotional upset is likely to show some diminution of REM period time, rather than an increase in it.

One minor corollary of Freud's theory of dream instigation was the proposition that dreams take place in an instant of time (the moment of awakening), in order to function as the "guardians of sleep." Freud was aware of the difficulty posed by the fact that dreams appear to last quite an interval of time. If they really did take place in an instant, one had to hypothesize a tremendous acceleration of the speed of thought-process in dreams, quite unlike anything in waking life. Freud was actually unsure how to solve this problem, but his tentative solution was to suppose that a dream "represents a fantasy which had been stored up ready-made in . . . memory for many years and which was aroused—or I would rather say 'alluded to' at the moment (1900, p. 496).

We now know that dreaming ordinarily occurs during a half-hour REM period, and, furthermore, that the apparent duration of a dream episode neatly coincides with the duration of REM activity. Dreaming episodes are thus clearly a concomitant of a physiological state, not a firework set off whenever sleep is threatened. But Freud's suggestion that dreams connect with stored affective memories and fantasies has had a very clear confirmation in REM studies, as we shall see in the next chapter.

The specific function that Freud theorized dreams as fulfilling was the discharge and healing of psychic wounds. In this sense, Freud's hypothesis about dreaming was that it was a sporadic affair—we dream when we are upset about something. Before the discovery of the regularly recurring REM period, therefore, the occurrence of a dream was an event that signified to most clinicians that some daytime conflict was at work. This theory of dreaming no longer holds—we dream during REM periods whether or not we are upset about something. Psychic wounds are not powerful enough to instigate a REM period, although this state may be used for some kind of physiological psychic and emotional discharge.

In fact, there is evidence that emotional arousal instigates dreaming *outside* REM periods. An interesting reversal of the general finding that there are more reports of dreaming from REM periods than from non-REM periods was obtained by Zimmerman (1967), who studied a group of "light" sleepers and "deep" sleepers in the laboratory. Among normal "light" sleepers (selected for their responsiveness to auditory-stimulus awakenings), 71% of non-REM awakenings yielded reports of dreaming, whereas only 21% of non-REM reports of "deep" sleepers yielded dream reports. During all their stages of sleep, the light sleepers had higher pulse rates, respiration rates, and body temperature than the deep sleepers. Along with their generally lower level of arousal, light sleepers appeared to be dreaming almost all night, a finding that suggests a connection between dreaming and arousal, but *outside* the REM period.

Like the biologically given functions of language and perception, the REM period occurs in all human beings regardless of their conflict state. It runs a developmental course from infancy to adulthood. At birth approximately 50% of sleep time is Stage 1 REMS; this amount decreases to 20% by age 3 or 4, continues at 20% until adulthood, and decreases further from age 50 to old age. Feeble-minded children have less REM time than normal controls (Feinberg, 1968). Ironically, therefore, dreaming is now a candidate for the list of "conflict-free" autonomous ego functions hypothesized by Hartmann!

The discovery of the REM period requires us to distinguish between dream episodes and dream content or experience. For the first time in history a biologically driven internal "clock" system has been uncovered as the major instigator for dream episodes. Freud's elaborate theory that the hallucinatory quality of dreams is the equivalent of the infant's first "hallucinatory wish"—that dream hallucinations are induced by emotional conflicts which create repression which in turn, together with sleep, creates a regressive backward flow of psychic energy over sensory pathways—is simply not tenable. It may be that *daytime* hallucinations of psychotic persons are sometimes induced by emotional conflict or repression, but ordinary dream episodes during the REMS are part of some general biological system.

The reader has probably already noted that the evidence against Freud's theory that dream episodes are triggered by emotional conflict is based upon an assumed equivalence between REM periods and dreaming. There is evidence, however, that dreaming experience and REM periods do not perfectly coincide. (Things could never be that simple!) On some occasions when they are awakened from REM periods, people will say that "nothing" was going through their minds, in other words, that they were not dreaming. On other occasions, people awakened from non-REM sleep will say that they have been having a dream. On many of the former occasions, no-dreaming reports are likely to have issued from REM periods earlier in the night—those occurring after deepest, or Stage 4, sleep (Goodenough, Lewis, Shapiro, Jaret, & Sleser, 1965). These first REM periods of the night are, in fact, shorter and less "busy" than succeeding episodes closer to morning. Thus it may be that they yield no-dream reports because the person has most recently been in a "sleep-fogged" physiological state which makes it harder to retrieve the content of dream experience.

As to the occasions when people say that they are dreaming out of a non-REM state, these reports are likely to occur during the transitions between sleeping and waking—either as hypnopompic or hypnagogic phenomena. These non-REM dream reports are, on the whole, qualitatively different from REM period dream reports in being less hallucinatory, more conceptual, and more often like "thoughts" about events of the preceding or coming day. A "blind" judge, using clearly defined criteria of whether an experience is "dreamlike" or "thoughtlike," was able to guess with reasonable accuracy whether a report had issued from a REM period or from a non-REM awakening (Shapiro, Goodenough, Lewis, & Sleser, 1965). These "thoughtlike" reports are thus often arousal phenomena. That is not to say that arousal phenomena are not sometimes extremely vivid and hallucinatory—for example, nightmares (with tachycardia and feeling of suffocation) issue out of Stage 4 non-REM sleep (Broughton, 1968), not out of REM periods as might have been assumed. But these are the relatively infrequent occasions when dreaming experience occurs outside a REM period. For the most part, the four cyclically recurring REM episodes that occur every night are accompanied by dreaming, and they occur with insistent regularity regardless of a person's emotional state. The preponderant equivalence between dreaming and REM periods is strong enough, therefore, to speak against Freud's theory of dream instigation.

In an effort to find support for that theory, some, including R. Jones (1974), have suggested that the mentation occurring during non-REM periods of sleep is the equivalent of Freud's "preconscious," out of which the dream forms during the REMS. But the existence of preconscious mentation during sleep, though it might help to explain the nature of dream content, cannot explain the regularly recurring instigation of dreaming during a physiological "third state."

Ironically, the observations of Silberer (1912/1951) and Federn (1952) that the hypnagogic and hypnopompic states foster transformations of daytime thoughts into symbolic dream imagery may be closer to the way things happen than Freud's idea that *all* dreams are instigated by emotional conflict.

A number of corollaries follow from the blow to Freud's theory about dream formation. The first of these is an alteration in the status of Freud's distinction between manifest and latent dream content. As we shall see in a moment, the distinction need not be abolished, but is important only in a restricted sense. A second, equally important corollary is an alteration of Freud's theory of dream recall and forgetting. Dream loss is no longer the result of repression alone. Still another corollary is an alteration in Freud's theory of the function of dreaming—his concept of the need to dream, and, specifically, of the dream as the "guardian of sleep." Each of these corollaries involves the destruction of the straitjacket that Freud had built around his observations about the meaning of dream content.

More than compensating this loss is an enormous gain in our ability to study dreams empirically, and to obtain some of the answers to the fascinating questions that Freud raised in the literature review with which he opened *The Interpretation of Dreams*. In addition, the problem of individual differences in dreaming style, which Freud did not address at all (since he was so busy establishing the fundamental meaning of dreams), can now be addressed.

Latent and Manifest Dream Content

One restricted meaning that has accrued to the concept of latent as opposed to manifest dreams remains unchanged by the discovery of the REMS. This is the notion of the uniqueness and individuality of the individual's stream of consciousness which is sampled in his dreams. The manifest content of a dream, like any other sample of thought, contains personal allusions to feelings and to biographical events that cannot be accurately identified without their unique connection to the individual's personal life. For example, a dream about the subway from a subway worker is a dream about his place of work as well as about a possibly symbolic element. Theoretically, as in this example, the individual's unique web of associations could be connected in a dream to a routine event as well as to conflict. But whether a dream is about conflict or about a trivial event may not be identifiable if we cannot correctly identify the references in the dream's content to the dreamer's personal life.

The logic of a theory postulating that conflict instigates dreaming did not permit the existence of any dream, however banal its appearance, that did not have connections to conflict, since by fundamental postulate, without conflict a dream would not have come into existence. Therefore, in Freud's theoretical system, the manifest content of a dream, even if it did not appear to reflect conflict, *had* to be connected with it. This line of reasoning was not only the result of some rigidity of thinking—some holding on to an "official position," as Erikson (1954) puts it—but also an outgrowth of a fundamental postulate.

The knowledge that conflict does not instigate all dreaming[2] releases the manifest content from the straitjacket of *necessary* connection to latent conflict which has encumbered it. Latent conflict may or may not inhere in manifest dreams.

The universal clinical observation that dream content is often about conflict may be understood by supposing that conflict is a prepotent stimulus at night, as it is during the day, and that ready-waiting dream time is likely to give it precedence over less potent stimuli. But in this model there is no intrinsic reason why relatively indifferent events may not also get into dreaming time. A contented person may have contented dreams, continuing his daytime psychic state. Mortal happiness is, however, "finely-checkered" (as Jane Austen puts it), so that the night's dreams of a contented person might pick up a few trivial grumbles. Since not every dream needs to plumb the psychic depths in order to justify its existence, the hallucinatory dream experience may be expressive of relatively trivial events, and in sleep-fogged, reduced intellectual level. The independent existence of dreaming aside from emotional disturbance thus releases the manifest content of dreams from *mandatory* translation as emotionally based and allows for the existence of dreams that straightforwardly represent ordinary or mundane life events. In this kind of instance, an attempt to connect each element of a

---

[2]Since we do not know what triggers the REM-period, the theoretical possibility remains that conflict is somehow indirectly involved in dream instigation. Furthermore, conflict, if it issues in arousal, may be the instigation of dreams occurring outside the REM period. In these instances it might be represented in the manifest content only in "disguise," that is, in "primary-process" transformation. But a theory of dreaming need no longer base itself on the assumption of a single cause for dreaming.

dream to a repression-connected source may be a mistranslation of the dream, which can be understood as more directly representing life experience. For example, a survey of the content of 635 REM period reports obtained from 58 young adults over 250 laboratory nights (Snyder, Karacen, Tharp, & Scott, 1967) concludes that dream reports are generally "clear, coherent, believable accounts of realistic situations in which the dreamer and other persons are involved—and usually talking about them." Snyder *et al.* thus find themselves in agreement with the characterizations of dreaming made by introspectionist psychologists who studied dreams at the turn of the century (and with whom Freud disagreed). That conflict is reflected even in "realistic" dreams is quite possible, but it is not axiomatic.

Clinicians must now learn to distinguish between dreams that express residues of mundane events and those that express emotionally significant events. Both trivial and emotionally significant dreams may occur in a manifest content that needs element-by-element breakdown and reassembly. But they both may also occur in dreams that can be understood symbolically or in gestalt fashion. It may be, for example, that people who use isolation of affect as a frequent defense cannot comprehend their dreams without a painstaking breakdown and reassembly, as we saw Freud do for his Irma dream. In other persons affects may be more generally visible both in their dreams and their waking lives.

Although Freud's theory of dream instigation was destroyed by the discovery of the REMS, his interpretation of some dream content (and forgetting) as transformations of forbidden affects is not damaged. Since the discovery of the REMS it has become possible to study these transformations in even greater detail than Freud could command, because we can now identify the actual occurrence of dream episodes and can retrieve their content on the spot. A much greater number of dreams is thus available to us for study—and even more important, it is possible for us to undertake systematic experimental manipulations of presleep emotional input, varying it from "neutral" to "conflictful." This line of research follows Silberer's and Nachmansohn's lead in its attempt to manipulate the presleep emotional experience. As we shall see in the next chapter, a large-scale study (Witkin & Lewis, 1965) has shown that translations of dreamers' presleep conflicts are recognizable in their dreams, using Freud's method of interpretation.

Repression and the Forgetting of Dreams

Freud's theory assumed that the same conflict forces that instigated a dream would also operate against its recall. Dream forgetting was thus intrinsically tied to repression, along with dream instigation and dream content. The discovery of the REMS also severs the supposed intrinsic connection between dream forgetting and repression.

Freud's impression that dreams are ephemeral experiences is, of course, confirmed by laboratory studies of dreaming, but the fragility of dreams seems to be a function of the sleep state in which they occur, not just of repression. Awakenings made only 5 minutes after the termination of a REM period, for example, will yield a significant loss in percentage of dream recall compared with awakenings made during the REM period itself (Goodenough et al., 1965). Considering that each of us has on the average about four REM periods in an ordinary 8-hour sleep, and that even the most gifted dream recallers among us remember one or at most two of their dreams of the night, it is fair to say that we routinely forget at least half if not the bulk of our dream experiences every night. The forgetting of dreams is thus a "normal" occurrence, for which repression cannot be a general explanation.

Before the discovery of the REMS, the recall of dreams was studied only as it happened on morning awakening. It was natural to assume that people who never or only rarely remembered their dreams were, by definition, "repressors," whereas people who regularly remembered their dreams were not users of this defense. This assumption was, of course, immediately called into question by the discovery that the great bulk of our dream life is normally lost to all of us. With the advent of laboratory studies of on-the-spot recall of dreams retrieved from REM periods, one of the first questions to be answered was whether dream recallers and dream forgetters differed in their REM periods. A study addressing this question showed clearly that when people sleep at home those who rarely recall their dreams are no different from the people who recall their dreams every morning in the number of their REM periods or in their EEG patterns (Goodenough, 1967; Lewis, Goodenough, Shapiro, & Sleser, 1966). And they continue to differ in their capacity to recall their dreams even in on-the-spot awakenings. Habitual dream recallers recall more dreams than do dream forgetters in the laboratory as well as at home. This finding once again encouraged the hypothesis that repression or some such personality characteristic is at work to explain the difference between dream recallers and forgetters.[3]

When we examined the content of their dreams in the hope of distinguishing in this way between "recallers" and "forgetters," there

[3]Since dream recall and dream reporting are not synonymous, it is probably more accurate to speak of dream reporters and nonreporters rather than recallers and forgetters. Using the terms "recallers" and "forgetters," however, highlights the issue being discussed, although the reader should bear in mind that the actual data are those of report and nonreport.

were no significant differences in the bizarreness or visual imagery of the dreams. Only one important characteristic of dream content was different between the two groups: the representation of the self in the dream. Those people who recalled their dreams at home had more dreams in the laboratory in which the self was the protagonist of the action. The memory function involved here seems to fit a familiar pattern. Better-organized material (in this case organized around the self as protagonist) is easier to remember. Simultaneously, however, this finding fits the notion that dream recallers and forgetters may have different organizations of the self. Specifically, people who have a less articulated sense of self are also likely to be field dependent; field-dependent people are also likely to make greater use of the defense of repression and denial. Finally, in this chain of connections, people who habitually do not recall their dreams (home nonreporters) are likely to be more field dependent than people who characteristically recall their dreams every morning (Bone, Thomas, & Kinsolving, 1972; Lewis *et al.*, 1966; Schonbar, 1965; Witkin, 1970). They are also more likely to be classified as repressors on personality tests (Robbins & Tanck, 1970; Singer & Schonbar, 1961; Tart, 1962). Since there is a connection between field dependence and characteristic use of repression and denial as defense, the picture clearly emerges of repression as an important factor in dream recall—but for particular personalities rather than as a general law. This is a line of inquiry that Freud never pursued since his theory required that *all* dream forgetting be the product of repression.

Laboratory studies of dream recall have also yielded some evidence that, as Freud predicted, anxiety can, on occasion, produce repression of dreams. The phenomenology of these occasions is extraordinarily like Freud's descriptions of the event. In contrast to REM period awakenings early in the night, after deep sleep, which yield reports that "nothing" was going through the person's mind, there are REM period awakenings in which a person says he was surely dreaming but just "lost" the dream—it was just "sucked away." But these accounts of dream loss, so reminiscent of how patients often describe their experience to therapists, are relatively infrequent in the laboratory. For example, in one study (Shapiro *et al.*, 1965) there were only 3 instances of such accounts in 160 awakenings. All three, however, were characterized by respiratory irregularity, suggesting that the dreams were particularly affectful ones and thus candidates for repression. Although a later study (Goodenough, Witkin, Lewis, Koulack, & Cohen, 1974) failed to confirm the finding that dreams accompanied by respiratory irregularity are more often lost on awakening, we did find that field-dependent individuals were more likely than field-independent people to "lose" the dreams that had been accompanied by stressful affect. This finding suggests that field-dependent people may be particularly prone to repress their anxiety-laden dreams. Repression, in other words, is not the single cause of dream forgetting, as Freud's theory required, but a description of dream loss as it occurs in some people.

The Need to Dream

Fairly soon after the discovery of the REMS came the evidence that REM periods are "imperative" happenings in a circadian rhythm. Deprivation of REM periods—that is, interruptions of REM periods before their completion—results in a "rebound" effect. People increase their REM period "attempts" by as much as 50% if they are deprived of their REM period sleep (Dement, 1969). This finding led to a formulation of a "need to dream," and was quickly equated with Freud's notion that dreams are "safety valves" for conflict or emotional expression.

In fact, Freud had theorized a very narrow meaning of the "need to dream." He hypothesized that the dream is instigated in order to protect the dreamer's sleep. In other words, Freud postulated a primary need to sleep—a need that physiologists have since shown us is on a level with need for food or water. Freud's "need to dream" was a by-product of this need to sleep. The question of what might happen to people if they were deprived of dreaming was not even considered by Freud. In human beings (as in cats and rats) the effect of REM deprivation seems to be an increase in cortical excitability, which suggests that some buildup of substances requiring discharge has taken place (Dement, 1969). But this is neurohumoral physiological discharge, not necessarily discharge of affect. The question whether there is a need for dreaming experience, and, if so, what function dreaming experience serves is a separate issue.

Since the discovery of the REMS, several theories have been advanced about its biological function. Snyder (1966), for example, has suggested that REM periods are a survival of the evolutionary value of an animal's alertness during sleep. Roffwarg, Muzio, and Dement (1966) have suggested that REM periods are feedback of endogenous stimulation that helps in the maturation of the central nervous system. Ephron and Carrington (1966) have suggested that REM episodes function to help the organism maintain some kind of cortical homeostasis during sleep's general slowdown of physiological functioning. All these hypothetical functions of the REMS attempt to understand the newly discovered biological "given."

As to the need for dreaming experience as distinct from the need for REM periods, the Freudian notion would presumably be that dreaming experience is needed in order to express emotional conflict. If there is a need for a completed dreaming experience (something like the Zeigarnik effect), as distinct from the need for REM periods, then the interruption of REM periods and the consequent inability to *complete* a dream should have different consequences from the simple loss of REM time through sleep deprivation. In fact, Sampson (1965) showed that interruption of REM periods (Dement's method) was no different in its effects on subsequent recovery nights than an equivalent amount of REM deprivation through sleep loss. Sampson interpreted his findings as speaking against a need for dream experience.

Other studies have shown that REM deprivation does have some effects on subsequent daytime behavior. Dement (1966) has shown that there are some noxious behavioral and personality consequences of REM deprivation, but no severe or irreversible personality damage. He also interprets his findings as speaking against a biological need for *dream experience.*

Still other studies have found that, at least for some people, REM period deprivation (resulting from REM interruption) does significantly affect the quality of subsequent dream content. Foulkes, Pivik, Ahrens, and Swanson (1968) found, for example, that those people with the greatest increase in REM-recovery time after REM interruption also showed a significant increase in the dreamlike quality or intensity of their dream experience.

There is evidence that field-dependent and field-independent subjects react differently to the effect of REM period deprivation. Cartwright, Monroe, and Palmer (1967) have shown that field-dependent subjects have their sleep cycle more disrupted by REM deprivation than field-independent subjects. In another study (Cartwright & Monroe, 1967) the effects of accompanying REM interruption with a brief repetitive task (reciting digits) were compared with the effects of telling dreams at REM interruption. Again, field-dependent subjects showed a greater effect of the digits-reciting condition on REM-recovery time, a result that was interpreted as indicating their greater need for dream experience. In these studies, field-dependence was determined by the figure-drawing test scored for sophistication of body concept.

Differences in cognitive style may also play a role in the individual's "need to dream" as reflected in the intensity of eye movement activity. Field-dependent subjects, for example, for reasons as yet unknown, have more eye movements during their REM periods than field-independent subjects (Lewis et al., 1966). Several different studies have shown that REM density is connected with the nature of dream content

(Lewis, 1970). Dreams characterized by a higher level of physical activity (Berger & Oswald, 1962; Dement & Wolpert, 1958; Lewis *et al.*, 1966), bizarreness, visual imagery (Lewis *et al.*, 1966), emotionality, aggression (Karacen, Goodenough, Shapiro, & Starker, 1966), or dream intensity (Pivik & Foulkes, 1966) are also characterized by more eye movements during the REM period from which they issue. It may be that field-dependent persons, who show more eye movements, may be transacting more "emotional business" in their dreams.

Lerner (1967) has postulated that dream content is needed for the expression of kinesthetic fantasy which, in turn, is needed for the reintegration of the body image. She showed (1966) that REM deprivation (effected by drugs) significantly increases the number of movement responses on the Rorschach test. Although she did not directly demonstrate an increase in kinesthetic fantasy in dream content after deprivation, Lerner has reviewed considerable evidence that compensatory kinesthesis plays an important role in dream content. This is in keeping with Rorschach's idea that kinesthetic fantasy (M) is antithetical to overt, gross motor activity. Berger (1967), working with monkeys, observed an inverse relationship between frequency of eye movements during waking activities and REM density in REM periods.

An inverse relationship between frequency of movement responses on the Rorschach test and field dependence has been observed (Witkin, 1965), and in a recent longitudinal study of Rorschach responses in relation to perceptual style, Schimek (1968) also found (indirect) evidence of a relationship between M scores and field dependence. It has also been established that field-dependent and field-independent persons differ in the degree of sophistication of the body concept. It might therefore be that field-dependent subjects, who ordinarily have fewer M responses on the Rorschach, and have a less developed body concept, would "need" more compensatory kinesthesis, and in turn, more eye movements in their dream periods. Some observations from my patients indicated that a field-dependent patient had more kinesthetic-visceral imagery in her dreams whereas a field-independent patient's dreams were more disembodied. As we shall see, this observation was also made in our film study.

In summary, then, the discovery of the REMS has significantly damaged Freud's theory of dream instigation, and with it, his concept of the unintelligibility of all manifest dream content, his concept of dream forgetting as the exclusive work of repression, and his concept of the "need to dream" in order to preserve sleep. But, as we shall see in the next chapter, Freud's interpretation of the emotional meaning of dream content remains extraordinarily useful.

CHAPTER 3

REMS Studies
The Problem of Tracing Emotions in Dream Content

We turn from Freud's theory of dream instigation to his interpretations of dream content as reflecting our emotional life. Here REMS studies offer fascinating examples of the power of emotional stimuli to invade dream content, and of the usefulness of Freud's translations of dream language into underlying affective content.

Laboratory studies have the disadvantage, however, of creating their own emotional complexities which may increase the difficulty of tracing specific emotional input into transformed dream content. One important finding in these studies is that differences in cognitive style are important determinants of the connection between emotional events and subsequent dream content. Another finding from REMS studies confirms the link between dream content and the content of early memories.

<small>ARE LABORATORY DREAMS REPRESENTATIVE OF DREAMS AT HOME?</small>

A first question that had to be answered, of course, was whether dreams obtained under laboratory conditions, and with elaborate EEG monitoring equipment on the person's body, would at all resemble dreams collected under the age-old conditions of morning awakening at

44

home. Observation from sleep laboratories suggested that they did, except that dreams in the laboratory were blander than dreams occurring at home. In many nights of observation, for example, few nightmares occurred in the laboratory. In one systematic study of home dreaming versus laboratory dreaming (Weisz & Foulkes, 1970), 12 young adult males spent two nonconsecutive nights at the laboratory and two at home, in counterbalanced order. They were awakened uniformly by an alarm clock at 6:30 A.M., and asked for dreams, if any. In ratings by "blind" judges, no differences were observed in the dreams obtained under the two conditions with respect to vivid fantasy, unpleasantness, active participation, and sex. Dreams at home were somewhat more aggressive in content than dreams in the laboratory. Weisz and Foulkes conclude that the basic dream processes of imagination, distortion, and dramatization are the same in both home and laboratory settings.

POTENCY OF EMOTIONAL STIMULI TO INVADE DREAMS

Freud's observation that dream content consists of material derived from emotionally important experience has been confirmed in a variety of REMS studies, some of them very imaginatively designed. For example, in a study of the psychophysiological correlates of dream content retrieved from REM awakenings, Hauri and VandeCastle (1970) found that the level of physical activity reported in a dream was *not* related to physiological arousal, whereas the emotionality of a dream and the extent of involvement of the person in it were significantly related to physiological arousal. In another approach to the role of emotions in dreaming, Hersch, Antrobus, Arkin, and Singer (1970) found that an injection of epinephrine during State 4 sleep (accomplished without waking the person) yielded dream reports, 10 minutes later, that were much more dreamlike—that is, significantly more imaginative, bizarre, vivid, emotional, and perceptual (as contrasted with conceptual)—than reports obtained after an injection of a saline solution. Clearly, autonomic—presumably emotional—arousal is followed by "dreamy" experience.

SOMATIC VERSUS EMOTIONAL SOURCES OF DREAM CONTENT

Freud remarked (in his *Introductory Lectures*, p. 238) that it is possible to influence what a person will dream about, but not *what* he will dream. Freud had observed that somatic stimuli, such as the sensations of "indigestion," could enter dream content, but he was convinced that this happened only when the somatic stimulus was also linked to emotional arousal. It will be remembered from Chapter 1 how Freud refused to allow painful boils to be the only source of his dream about riding a horse: The theme itself was also a metaphor for feelings of humiliation that Freud had experienced in connection with one of his patients.

The discovery of the REMS had made it possible experimentally to vary somatic stimuli during or immediately preceding REM periods, and to examine subsequent dream content for the appearance of each particular stimulus. Many findings suggest that Freud was right in his insistence on the importance of emotional rather than strictly somatic stimuli. Experimental studies have shown, in the first place, that visual, auditory, and tactile stimuli offered during the REM period (without waking the person) do not easily enter into immediately retrieved dream content. Dement and Wolpert (1958), for example, found that a pure tone made it into dreams in 9% of trials offered; a visual stimulus in 23% of trials; and a drop of water in 42% of the trials. Tactile stimuli are thus more potent than either visual or auditory stimuli, but none of these stimuli was very potent to influence dream content.

If, however, the auditory stimulus has some emotional meaning—for example, a personal name—then it is incorporated into subsequent dream content (Berger, 1963). The subjects in Berger's experiment were four men and four women students. A tape played the name of a girl friend or a boyfriend as the subject entered the REMS, or else it played a "neutral" personal name. Twenty seconds later the subject was awakened and asked for content, if any. The dreamer, as well as an independent judge, was asked to match the dream to the stimulus that had been fed into the REMS. Contrary to prediction, there was no difference in the *frequency* with which neutral and emotional names were perceived in dream content. But both kinds of stimuli were transformed in the subject's dreams, in a way that closely resembles Freud's description of "dream work" and Ella Sharpe's description of metaphors in dreams (cf. Chapter 1). For example, names were most frequently incorporated by assonance, and also by associative links and by visual representation. There were also several instances of sexual symbolism in the dreams and these occurred only after the name of the subject's boy or girl friend.

Another ingenious experiment compared the effects of exposure to a tape of one's own voice during the REMS with the effects of another person's speaking the same words (Castaldo & Holzman, 1967). There were more dreams in which the protagonist took an active, independent, and assertive role after exposure to his or her own voice during the REMS than after exposure to someone else's voice. In the latter condition, the dream's protagonist was more often passive. Castaldo and Holzman interpret their finding as dependent upon a link between hearing one's own voice and "voluntary action." Although dreams with an active protagonist do not necessarily represent any more or less affect than dreams with a passive one, it is clear that the affective component of a stimulus is a significant determinant of a dream's content and in an appropriate or at least understandable way.

Still another line of experiment has systematically varied the individual's actual somatic state in relation to dream content. Bokert (1968) found that subjects who had been deprived of fluids and given a salty meal before sleep had more references to thirst in their dreams than nondeprived people. He also found that people whose dreams explicitly gratified thirst were actually less thirsty and drank less on awakening than people who did not have explicit thirst gratification in their dreams. This finding coincides with a finding (Domhoff & Kamiya, 1964) that references to food and drink normally increase during the course of the dreams of the night, as an apparent result of the buildup of these needs during sleep. Dreams thus do express the gratification of "wishes," and not just in children and geese!

The discovery that erections of the penis are a regular part of the REM period suggests that Freud's observations about the prominence of sexual conflict in dreaming may have been a most inspired guess. Freud (1900) observed that the majority of symbols in dreams are sexual in nature and that they are translated "at sight" (p. 153). The sexual organ arousal during the REMS may help account for this content. Although the physiologists have rightly pointed out that penile erections during sleep represent physiological arousal and do not necessarily indicate sexual experience, it is clear that physiological arousal of the sexual organs is an undercurrent of our dreams. (Analogous clitoral arousal during the REMS has been observed in women.) And although there is no clear way to separate the physiological and psychological components of this recurrent stimulus during sleep, one line of investigation has shown that REM periods in which there is slight, variable, or absent penile erection are also those in which dream content is characterized by a high level of anxiety (Karacen et al., 1966). The linkage between anxiety and loss of erection which Freud first observed as "castration anxiety" is thus clearly visible in men's dreams.

It is interesting to note, in passing, that the existence of penile erections during the REMS has suggested a basis for the differential diagnosis of organic versus psychophysical sexual impotence. In patients with psychogenic impotence, performance when awake was observed to be markedly inferior to their nocturnal erections during the

REMS, whereas in organic cases no such discrepancy occurred (C. Fisher, Schiavi, Lear, Edwards, Davis, & Witkin, 1975).

DREAMING AND PSYCHOSIS

In line with the reasoning that dreams are about emotional disturbance, Freud had remarked that dreams are like a nightly psychosis. This observation actually had been made by earlier writers, many of whom Freud quoted. Kant is quoted as saying that "the lunatic is a wakeful dreamer"; Hughlings Jackson, Freud's contemporary, had said: "Find out about dreams and you will find out about insanity." And Jung, Freud's follower in the beginning of his work, had said: "Let the dreamer walk about and act like one awakened and we have a clinical picture of dementia precox."

REMS studies of the sleep and dreaming of depressed and schizophrenic patients have yielded results which suggest that a difference in affect management can be distinguished in their dreams. One of the first questions studied after the discovery of the REMS was that of the dreaming of schizophrenics. Advance predictions had suggested that schizophrenics might have no "dream time" at all since they "did their dreaming" while awake. Dement (1955) was the first to undertake a comparison of the sleep of schizophrenics and normals and found no striking differences. His findings have been subsequently confirmed (Feinberg, Koresko, & Gottlieb, 1965). Dement did observe, however, that the content of schizophrenics' dreams was different from normals in only one respect: that it contained isolated, inanimate objects about which nothing was happening. Half of the schizophrenic patients had dreams with these isolated, single images, but this phenomenon was entirely absent from the dreams of normal medical-student controls. The relative absence of distinguishing dream content in schizophrenia was also found in a study by Richardson and Moore (1963), who collected dreams on morning recall at home. They found that 15 experienced psychiatrists and psychoanalysts were not able to distinguish between the dreams of schizophrenics and matched normal controls.

In contrast, REMS studies of dreaming in depressives have yielded significant differences from normals in sleep cycle as well as in dream content. Even without using the REMS Beck and his coworkers (1967) found that severely depressed psychotic patients had manifest dreams that differed significantly from those of less depressed patients, specifically in increased "masochistic" content. Clinical improvement, however, contrary to expectation, brought no corresponding change in dream content. (It is interesting to note that Beck has since espoused a cognitive as opposed to a psychoanalytic theory of depression.)

The depressed patient takes longer to fall asleep, has more wakefulness during sleep, wakes earlier in the morning, and has less of Stage 4 (deep) sleep as well as less time spent in Stage 1. (That depressives have less REM time is a general finding, but on some occasions they may show a rebound effect and exhibit more REM time.) But the most consistent and persistent abnormality is that they have a diminution or absence of Stage 4 sleep (E. Hartmann, 1969). Depressives' clinical complaint of "poor sleep" is amply confirmed by the characteristics of their sleep cycle. In addition, the content of their dreams retrieved from monitored REM periods is significantly "depressed." In one study (Kramer, Whitman, Baldridge, & Lansky, 1966), for example, depressed patients had more dreams with Beck's "masochism" themes, and more dreams with themes of helplessness, hopelessness, and of "escape and suicidal wishes" than appeared in the dreams of normals.

This difference between the clearly discernible masochistic content of the dreams of depressed patients and the relative absence of "trademarks" in the dreams of schizophrenics may itself be a function of the difference between those two functional disorders in their mode of affect management. Affective disturbance is to the fore in depression in contrast to affective shutdown in schizophrenia, and this characteristic difference may also be distinguishable in dreams.

Thus, in summary, a variety of experiments using REM monitoring techniques have shown emotional stimuli to be potent infiltrators of dreams. Perhaps the best way of illustrating the hardiness of Freud's methods of dream interpretation is to examine some of the dreams and dreaming phenomena observed in the laboratory as a consequence of emotional arousal.

TRANSFORMATIONS OF EXPERIMENTALLY INDUCED EMOTIONAL STRESS IN DREAM CONTENT

I come now to a large-scale study of the effects of experimentally induced presleep emotional arousal on subsequent dreams in which I was a collaborator, along with H. A. Witkin, Donald Goodenough, and Arthur Schapiro, and others over a number of years. A fuller account of the procedure and some results of this study may be found in Witkin and Lewis (1967) and Witkin (1970). In this study we based ourselves on Freud's observation that emotional upset (anxiety) is a prepotent stimulus in invading dreams. For the most part we used short emotionally charged and neutral films as our presleep stimuli. As stress films we used Roheim's film of subincision initiation rites among the Arunta and a film showing the birth of a baby. Our neutral films were two travelogues, one about London and the other about the American far west.

Subincision Film

This is a film made by Geza Roheim of a rite practiced by an aboriginal Australian group, the Arunta. (These are the people who figure in Freud's *Totem and Taboo*, 1913.) It shows a number of older men preparing for the initiation of four young men. All the men are naked. Each initiate in turn lies down across the backs of the other initiates, who are perched on all fours close to each other, creating a "table" or "couch" for the operation. An incision is made along the ventral surface of the penis with a sharp stone. The bleeding penis is then seen being held over a smoking fire. The faces of the initiates clearly reveal their anguish. A hairdressing ritual is shown. The film ends with a rhythmic ritual dance by the initiates, resumably after their recovery from the incision. The Roheim film has been used by others, notably Lazarus, Speisman, Mordkoff, and Davison (1962), as a stimulus for the evocation and measurement of stress.

Birth Film

This is a medical teaching film in color, prepared at Downstate Medical Center. It begins with a description of the Malmstrom Vacuum Extractor and discusses its advantages as a method of delivery. The next part shows the exposed vagina and thighs of the woman, painted with iodine. The arm of the obstetrician is seen inserting the vacuum extractor into the vagina; the gloved hands and arms of the obstetrician are then shown pulling periodically on a chain protruding from the vagina. The cutting motion of the episiotomy is also shown. The baby is then delivered with a gush of blood. The film ends by illustrating that only a harmless swelling of the skin of the baby's head results from the vacuum-extraction method.

We expected that dreams after a stressful film would be recognizably different in their content from dreams after a neutral film, and also that the "loss" (repression) of dream content would occur more often after stress than after neutral films. We also postulated that the effects of emotionally exciting events would be greater for field-dependent than for field-independent people, and that field-dependent people would "lose" their dreams after stress more often than field-independent people. As I have already indicated, we did confirm this last prediction (Goodenough et al., 1974). We also found that, as predicted, subjects reported more anxiety after seeing the stress films than after neutral films, and that the content of their subsequent dreams was more anxious as measured by the Gottschalk-Gleser method of assessing verbal productions for implied affect (Gottschalk-Gleser, 1969). But, anticipating our story a bit, we found that our predictions about the effects of stress and neutral films on dream content were made difficult to pursue by the unexpected "interference" of an emotional relationship between the experimenter and the subject that developed in the course of a 6-week study, as well as by a carry-over from the exciting film into the next week's officially neutral session. Probably as a result of these factors we were not able to obtain "blindly guessed" differences in dream content after our stress and neutral films. This outcome parallels the findings of Foulkes and Rechtschaffen (1964) that judges could not guess from dream texts which film, an exciting western or a quieter romantic film, had preceded sleep. But we did obtain a wealth of evidence attesting to the vitality of Freud's descriptions of the "dream work." In this respect our findings parallel those of Berger (1963), who also failed to obtain a difference between emotional and neutral names in the frequency of incorporation but found evidence for the "dream work" as the means of incorporation.

SYMBOLIC TRANSFORMATIONS IN DREAMS: COGNITIVE STYLES

The wealth of evidence for the usefulness of Freud's descriptions of the dream work can also be glimpsed even from a few excerpts of the transcripts of dreams retrieved from REM awakenings after our stress films. Understandable symbolic transformations of castration and homosexuality themes were in abundance after the subincision film; likewise, pregnancy and childbirth symbols occurred after the birth film. For example, after the subincision film, there were dreams containing such generally recognized castration and homosexual symbols as: an airplane crash; blindness; having a flat tire; broken glasses; holding a floppy rubber scoop; being a captive; going over Niagara Falls; two men biting each other's back. Each example I have cited comes from a different dream text after the subincision film and all but the first two come from different subjects. Similarly, after the birth film themes of penetration, pregnancy, womb, and birth were apparent in transformation in the dream content: for example, being on a crowded bus; putting slugs in boxes; a woman in a smock; an old kitchen sink (with the inscription, "A woman's toil is never done"); reaching for a gun on a shelf; being in a small kitchen; a huge grapevine; a little girl stumbling and falling down; picking peaches at a vegetable stand.

In order to convey, as well, the flavor of the stylistic differences between our field-dependent and field-independent subjects, I have selected excerpts from two subjects, one at each end of the field-independence continuum.

Let us look first at the dreams after the subincision film of Subject 25, a field-dependent black man, 28 years old, married, father of two children, a subway porter who had been trained as a welder but had been unable to join the closed union in that field of work.

> I don't . . . I don't think I was dreaming anything. I seem to have some sort of picture of water running down a gutter. And that seemed to be all . . . Was nobody around . . . No, it was different . . . It was acetyline hoses . . . being used for draining . . . For like . . . they were red and green . . . And I *got my feet wet . . . But I couldn't see myself.*

Adding one further detail to the dream text, the subject said that he "didn't know where the hoses were attached to" but that there was an acetyline hose and an oxygen hose (as is appropriate in the welding process). The two italicized elements in the subject's dream report reflect that he has had a kinesthetic experience. The acetyline hoses are relatively mundane images, since they are in actual use in welding.

In the postsleep inquiry into his experiences, Subject 25 explained to the experimenter that acetyline and oxygen hoses are used in connection with acetyline torches. It was clear that this was a technical detail of welding of which the experimenter was ignorant. In describing the events of the subincision film in his own words, this subject said: "They didn't seem to know what they were doing . . . they didn't know technology. They weren't in the know." In the midst of his telling this dream, there developed a lengthy discussion between subject and experimenter of the former's resentment at discrimination against blacks, especially in the union he was unable to enter. The technical detail about acetyline hoses can thus be understood as an oblique reference to the subject's resentment—a feeling that was also evoked by his watching the subincision film (about blacks) shown to him by a white experimenter.

The hoses are also interpretable as a symbolic transformation of the penis. Asked by the experimenter whether this dream element might be connected with the film, the subject replied as follows:

SUBJECT: I don't think so. These hoses are real narrow.
EXPERIMENTER: They were narrow?
SUBJECT: Yeah, and very long . . .
EXPERIMENTER: Well, you say they're narrow, and therefore it didn't have
    anything to do with it. What if they were . . . not narrow?
SUBJECT: I don't think it had anything to do with it.
EXPERIMENTER: No. I was just trying to understand . . .
SUBJECT: They were . . . narrow and long. Long. And that wouldn't have
    anything to do with the penis or anything. To me.

We thus repeat here the familiar observation of Freud that symbolic representations of sexual symbols are not recognizable by the dreamer although they may be obvious to anyone else.

Another element in this dream after the subincision film was the subject's kinesthetic image of getting his feet wet. In describing his very earliest memory, the subject (who was raised in an orphanage) remembers that he was "very little." "And there was water . . . I was told not to go near it." Once again, the water in his dream—which could symbolically represent the bleeding shown in the film—is also specifically connected in his early memory to a "no-no." "If it had been me," said Subject 25, commenting on the film, "first place I don't ever think they'd have got me. I'da been fighting like hell." The theme of getting his feet wet when he was told not to, derived from his earliest childhood, thus connects with and represents his resentment at authority, but in a relatively passive mode.

After the birth film, Subject 25 dreamed that he was

> riding on the subway . . . and a lady was selling raisin bread. And the
> subway wasn't moving. But . . . the lady had kind of . . . some new kind of
> bread. But I didn't see no raisins . . . The bread had no crust . . . And this
> lady with a cart, selling raisin bread.

This dream, following the birth film, contains symbolic breast imagery. And, as we shall see later in this chapter, the imagery of the dream and of this subject's earliest childhood recollection are remarkably similar in feeling. In the postsleep session the subject added some details of this dream. He said he had seen the "cellophane," a detail he had not mentioned in his immediate post-REM dream account. He also said that the bread appeared to him to be in an incubator—that the cart from which the bread was being sold was like an incubator, and he spontaneously related this additional imagery to the birth film. It then developed on inquiry that he had seen such an incubator when visiting his wife after the delivery of their premature baby! Thus emotionally charged experiences are condensed in his dream about raisin bread being sold by a woman.

Subject 14 is a field-independent white man, 29 years old, a factory worker, also married and the father of two children. At his first awakening after the subincision film, Subject 14 reported very little content, except that "it's a bad dream." Some 9 months later, in the course of a biographical interview, when asked to associate to the words "bad dream," Subject 14 said:

> Mummy. Mummy. M-u-m-m-y. Not Mommy. Mummy. That's from when I was a kid. I went—my mother told me not to go to see this picture *The Mummy's Hand* . . . and uh . . . I had terrible dreams about it. It was a frightening picture. I musta been, well, I hadda be under 7 when I saw it. And I was frightened to death. [This subject's mother died when he was 7 years old.] She warned me not to go see it and I went, and I was screaming for her . . . I was in the *bedroom* . . . and she said, "I'm not coming up there." (italics added)

At his third awakening, Subject 14 had dreams involving his mother-in-law, of whom he was a bit scornful, especially over her "putting on airs." (He perceived his mother-in-law as something of a Mrs. Malaprop.) At the third awakening, the subject had a very cheerful dream that he was about to go fishing when suddenly he was standing in his children's *bedroom* with his arm around his mother-in-law's waist, "swinging her around." He "felt her." The subject's earliest memory is of rolling in some puddles in a new suit, getting severely whacked for it and dumped naked into his crib, where he was left crying for a long time. Once again, therefore, there is a connection between his memory of screaming for his mother—in his *bedroom*—and his jolly, sexy dream which rights an old injury! He is now in his children's bedroom, swinging his mother-in-law around.

The subject's fourth dream is about a couple who are in business with a casting machine "equipped with a big grinding wheel" and including an "old silver trophy" that some man is grinding down; all the "grindings go down on a couch-like," and the man is boasting that he is doing this as a modernization—"modernizing things."

The subject's own words in describing the subincision film contain the elements that appear in his fourth dream. He picked up a detail of the film in which it seemed to him "as if they were sharpening stones or something." This is represented in the image of a grinding machine. Even more important, the subject had said that the experimenter's showing him the film was "outrageous. You know, it got me mad for a second . . . Why should they show this goddamn thing." The subject's dream in which he ridicules a couple with their modernizing machine can be understood as a retaliating, ridiculing reference to the experimenter's strange business, and in an active mode of aggression against the experimenter. It is also possible to interpret the "old silver trophy," which the subject described as V-shaped, comparing it to the "hood emblems for an old Packard," as the dream's representation of the incised penis, which does indeed present a V-shape after the incision is made.

Two of Subject 14's dreams after the birth film had images of seeing himself and other men kidding women, as he and the other men sat around watching movies together. Only at one awakening was Subject 14 at a loss for dream content: He could say only that his dream involved "having something to eat." During the postsleep inquiry the subject volunteered to tell the experimenter that he had actually recalled much more of this dream as he went back to sleep, but had decided not to ring the experimenter to report the addendum. The transcript of the subject's account again gives us the flavor of how piecemeal and often hesitant is the recall of emotionally charged, "repressed" material.

> Right after we, I, hung up, I started, you know, get little pieces back and it was this where I said I was eating? Did I say? [Experimenter: "Uh-huh."] There was this break, like a break wagon, break, the wall was full of these machines. Not break machines that you've seen before. They were open, everything was out in the open and there were, there were slots in the wall and then down the bottom you could take it out, the potato chips, like. And it was all along this wall . . . you just put your money in like I said and slide it down, take it out . . . you could steal it . . . it was just laying on the wall and you could rip the bag and take it away without paying . . . I was just about to buy a bag of potato chips and I . . . you know it was so vivid that when you rang the buzzer I put the stuff I had in my hands down . . . I just put the stuff right down here. Like I had it in my hand.

In describing his reactions to the birth film, the subject remarked that his wife had taken a book out of the library about childbirth and was amazed that they "allowed it on the shelves." He was aware, in other words, of the illicit quality of viewing women's exposed genitalia. The connection between seeing a "forbidden" film about childbirth and having a dream in which he "rips the bag" of food out of a machine in which everything "was out in the open" rests on an early memory of being punished in his mouth for taking something forbidden into his mouth. Subject 14 remembered that his mother had washed out his mouth with Kirkman's soap because he had picked up a cigarette butt. (This must also have been before he was 7, which was his age when his mother died.) That his dream was about getting some food can be understood as a symbolic equation between food and women. Subject 14 spontaneously commented that his dreams of this session were full of food and women, in a detached self-observation that is characteristic of field-independent people.

We come, finally, to a series of happenings in the laboratory experience of Subject 14 that illustrate how our neutral films were often overshadowed by feelings that developed toward the experimenter and toward the experimental situation itself. During the showing of the London film, which in this instance followed the subincision film that so outraged him, Subject 14 had a dream within a dream about a girl who was supposed to produce an erection in him and did! She was "something you [the experimenter] brought into the act . . . I think I was yelling to you . . . well you got the reaction." Asked what was going through his mind when he was viewing the London film the subject said that he "was wondering what you expected." Furthermore, the subject had during the week had a rather heated discussion (obviously initiated by himself) with fellow workers about whether or not it was "weird" to allow oneself to be a subject in such an experiment. One of the men at work had asked "would you let them watch you get a hard-on or something like this so this guy says you give me 15 [the subject's fee for participation], you can go into the shop with me . . . and see me get a hard-on." The subject wanted the experimenter's opinion about who was right, the subject or the men who were ridiculing him. The experimenter had some trouble dodging the issue.

In addition, the subject had told his wife his dream about her mother. His wife had interpreted his dream as follows:

> that because of the film, that puberty rite, and I don't have my own mother, my mother passed away, that I was asking her mother for protection so this wouldn't happen to me. This is how her and her girl friend analyzed that dream. This girl friend's husband says that dream was because I wanted because I was in the kids' bedroom and there was no kids, I wanted to get rid of the kids . . . my mother-in-law was just a woman then . . . and I just wanted my mother-in-law as a woman.

Once again, the subject tried to engage the experimenter in deciding between these two interpretations, and the experimenter had trouble handing the question back to the subject.

Needless to say, with such an arousal carried over from the preceding week, the subject's dreams after seeing the London Film were full of symbols of castration and homosexuality such as might be expected after the subincision film. It was clearly still uppermost in his mind.

The two interpretations of the subject's "mother-in-law" dream by his wife and a male friend of theirs are both a measure of how Freudian understanding of the emotional basis of dreams has become a part of household wisdom. The wife's interpretation is gentler, and catches more of her husband's anxiety; the male friend's interpretation prefers sexual arousal to anxiety as the mainspring. It is again a measure of the vitality of Freud's observations that the two explanations can be combined in the realization that (guilty) sexual arousal often functions to relieve (shameful) anxiety, as may have happened in this instance.

THE EFFECT OF HYPNOTIC SUGGESTION AS A PRESLEEP EXPERIENCE

We were also aware that our subjects must be responding not only to the particular films we showed them, but also to the laboratory situation itself. The experimenter, who is the "master of ceremonies," is particularly salient in creating another wide variety of experiences, some affecting the subject's dignity as well as, very literally, his body. In order to pursue this line of stimulus incorporation more directly we devised a simple "suggestion" session as a presleep stimulus that presumably would heighten the experimenter–subject interaction and highlight the subject's mode of dealing with this source of emotional arousal. In our original experimental plan we had thought that we might compare the effects of brief hypnotic suggestion with the effects of a film viewing, but the content analysis of the hypnotic suggestion experience seemed intrinsically so different that we thought it best to use films for our systematic comparison of stress and neutral experiences. We did, however, do a pilot experiment with hypnotic suggestion as our stimulus, retrieving dreams from subsequent REM periods. We envisaged the hypnotic suggestion session as a form of invasion—however mild—into the subject's self-boundaries.

The suggestion session took place after the subject was "hooked up" for EEG monitoring, and began with a discussion of people's bodily experiences. For example, the subject was asked what body position he prefers when falling asleep; for any unusual body sensations that precede sleep; how easily he falls asleep. He was then asked if he would be willing to try a few standard suggestion tests (which, in fact, they are) to check on an idea we had that people are more suggestible when they are drowsy. For a 2-minute period, the repetitive suggestion was made that the subject's right hand was getting heavier and warmer than his left hand. At the end of 2 minutes, he was asked to compare the sensations in his two hands. The suggestion was then repeated for another 2 minutes, and then another suggestion was then repeated for another 2 minutes, and then another suggestion was offered, namely, that the subject would find it difficult to take his clasped hands apart. At the end of this 2-minute period, the subject was asked to check on how difficult it was to take his hands apart. The subject then went to bed, and following our usual procedure, was awakened at each succeeding REM period.

Although the suggestions we used were very mild, they did "take" for our subjects. Here is a partial transcript of the dream retrieved from the spontaneous awakening of one subject. This transcript is presented in some detail as a sample of the way in which the content of the person's dream (delivered in a drowsy state) makes its appearance piecemeal, as the person struggles to retrieve it from sleep.

> SUBJECT: Well there was, there was a tune that was constantly running through my head and uh . . . I . . . I was thinking that I was half useful or that I was half connected. I had a dream during this period that I had my right arm in a sling. My right arm, and uh people were coming to visit me, and that I was only able to do half as much as I could normally do. That's uh . . . that was it. That was the one and only dream which I have had.
>
> EXPERIMENTER: You say there were people coming to visit?
>
> SUBJECT: Yes, uh, it was very brief . . . oh, oh, I don't know. It must have been about ten seconds . . . Uh, seems they were walking on one side of the street, and they were coming to visit me, and I had uh . . . I was only half useful. Everything seemed to be in half. And I had one of my arms in a sling . . . I believe it was the right arm.
>
> EXPERIMENTER: Everything seemed to be in half?
>
> SUBJECT: Uh, people were walking on one half of the street, and I . . . with one arm in a sling, was the other half of the street. Things were sectioned off in halves. Yeah.
>
> EXPERIMENTER: And where was this taking place?
>
> SUBJECT: I don't think it was any particular place. It could have been right outside here . . . in front of the building.
>
> EXPERIMENTER: It was outside of the building?
>
> SUBJECT: I'm not even sure. I'm not even sure. I know there were one . . . people were walking in single file. I'd say on one side of the street and I, with my arm in a sling, was on the other side of the street. If it was outside at all, that I . . . I don't remember.
>
> EXPERIMENTER: Did you recognize any of the people?
>
> SUBJECT: No. No . . . it was just uh . . . it was even . . . like I said I was in one half of the picture and these people were one behind the other in single file . . . in the other half of the picture. I didn't recognize anybody. They were evenly spaced, one in back of the other.
>
> EXPERIMENTER: And what about you? Were you doing anything?
>
> SUBJECT: No, I . . . I just had my arm in a sling, and I think I might have been walking in the same direction as they were walking. It was very brief. I don't even know if it was a dream. It might have been just a feeling or a thought that I was only half useful.
>
> EXPERIMENTER: And how did you feel during this?
>
> SUBJECT: Uh, I think that was when I first, uh . . . I first had to go to the john. I might have been lying on my side . . . and I wasn't uh . . . I wasn't let's see using my full capacity. Half of me uh was . . . was . . . somewhere else. I think I was going to the bathroom . . . something like that.

How I had my arm in a sling I don't know. I don't know how that ties in. It
was a brief, very brief passing thought.
EXPERIMENTER: And then you said there was a tune going through your
head?
SUBJECT: Yeah. Uh . . . should I hum it for you?
EXPERIMENTER: Okay . . . would you?
SUBJECT: Okay (hums; then sings) "You Took Advantage of Me" (hums
again) That's the one.

The subject's presleep experience of being subjected by the experimenter to effective suggestions about the right side of his body is clearly
represented in this dream by the "loss" of that side of the body. Even
more striking, the bodily feeling of being in half is projected onto the
world, resulting in a physiognomic perception of "things" being in half,
encompassing both the body and the field. The visitors "evenly spaced"
may have picked up the repetitive quality of the experimenter's suggestions. The whole scene evoked by the dream is of a Kafkaesque
world, "in half," in which the person has "lost" his accustomed self.

But perhaps the most dramatic feature of the dream's transformations of affects is its punch line: "You Took Advantage of Me." The
subject was apparently unaware of any feeling of hostility toward the
experimenter, even though he had wondered whether the experimenter
was trying to hypnotize him without being honest about it. By the time
the whole sleep session was over, the subject had quite forgotten the
title of the song. It is possible to speculate that by forgetting it he was
able to avoid expressing the feeling in it to the experimenter in a face-to-
face encounter. When he was asked if he thought the title of the song
had any connection with the suggestion session, he saw no connection.

Another of this subject's dreams in the same sleep session had
many images of violence and brutality: a bullet being removed from
someone; his car (which he owned jointly with his father) being demol-
ished—"ripped apart."

The dreams of other subjects after the suggestion session also contained many prominent references to the body, but in rather different
style from the preceding subject's dreams. Two other subjects had clas-
sic embarrassment dreams. Central in these dreams was the experience
of being watched in an awkward state—in one case, the subject was
urinating publicly in an elevator; another subject dreamed that he was
slipping on a banana peel as the shabby hero of a "very small parade,"
and then was being carried off in a horsecart. Both of these men were
openly resentful that the suggestion had worked. Their dreams reflect
the chagrin of this waking experience in the more fully developed dream
scenes of embarrassment and ridicule.

HYPNAGOGIC REVERIE STUDY

Another line of inquiry we pursued was into the stream of consciousness as a person is falling asleep following emotional arousal (Bertini *et al.*, 1964). We also retrieved the content of the first following dream, with the idea of tracing emotional arousal as it is transformed during the hypnagogic state and in the subsequent dream state. For this study we employed a combination of "white noise" and a visual "Ganzfeld" as the means of fostering the hypnagogic state. On some occasions we showed people an emotionally arousing film before they entered into the hypnagogic state and subsequent sleep.

A look at the transcript of one subject will illustrate how transformations proceed using not only simile and metaphor but also associative links that connect imagery and ideation with the person's still salient emotional memories. The transcript comes from the hypnagogic reverie previously cited in Chapter 1. The subject had just seen a film showing a mother monkey eating her dead baby. (This is a silent film in black and white made in the Primate Laboratory of the State University of New York Downstate Medical Center by Drs. I. Kaufman and L. Rosenblum.) The mother monkey is shown hauling the dead infant around by its arms and legs and nibbling at it. There are many scenes of the dangling legs of the dead baby.

Mr. A's last reported image as he was falling asleep was of a frog in a pool of clear water, a "blue-green frog with dark gray spots." It was, as he later remembered, a vivid visual image, "as if it were before me." Mr. A's choice of a frog to represent seeing a baby would be interpreted by Freud symbolically: A frog is a small animal; so is a baby. A frog also lives in a pool, jumping in and out, and it is usually brown—all qualities that connect it by simile and metaphor to fecal matter. Frog is thus an anal image of a baby, as well as connected to baby via the similarity in both being small animals. But Mr. A's use of frog was also apparently determined by unique association to his own experience with frogs. He remembered that he used to be "cruel" to frogs when he was a boy: He would throw them across a brick-wall incinerator and kill them. (One might speculate that they symbolically represented babies for him.) "After a while frog hunting became a little scarce. I suppose they *ran away* when they saw me" (italics added). The "frog" in the hypnagogic reverie is thus connected with guilty recollections of his own cruelty. Mr. A's first image is his subsequent dream is of "someone *being chased*" (as the guilty deserve to be).

In his second REM awakening, Mr. A reported the following dream: "I was staring into a large pail of water . . . in the water were what looked like three shrimp, one dark colored and very big and two light-colored ones." "Shrimp" is, of course, slang for a small child or baby. Mr. A said further that one shrimp looked like a grasshopper. Frogs, shrimps, and grasshoppers all have prominent legs; they are also all anal images. And perhaps even more compelling as an interpretation is the theme of Mr. A's guilt toward fish as well as frogs. Mr. A remembered that he used shrimp as bait on a fishing trip some years ago. When the fish died on that occasion, he "threw them back into the water and the seagulls came along and had a free lunch." Mr. A said, further, that he did not like to look at shrimp, especially when they were raw, because "when they're alive they don't look so good, all *legs*" (italics added). Mr. A's reverie had, in fact, contained many references to seagulls—which in this instance represent the cannibalistic theme in the movie, and quite specifically in resonance with Mr. A's guilt about animals that one eats.

Dreams and Early Memories

Freud observed that dream content represents feelings stirred during the day and still active at night because linked to repressed, "indestructible" wishes. Memories stored by a person as his earliest or early recollections were interpreted as "screen memories" covering powerful feeling states experienced in the past. Screen memories were summoned into dreams by "allusion." On this basis there should be an observable connection between the content of dreams and the recollections of childhood. It should be noted in passing that an important development in psychoanalytic thinking has been the use of early memories as a diagnostic indicator, both of pathology (Langs, 1965) and of personality (Mayman, 1968). Mayman has developed a test for proneness to shame or guilt using a person's early memories.

A direct connection was observed between the content of the dreams after the films and the content of the subject's earliest childhood recollections. The verbal similarity of content reported in the dream experience and the subject's earliest memory was sometimes striking enough so that little or no inference was needed to establish the connection. In other instances, the establishment of similarity in content required some steps of inference. A theme of the earliest childhood recollection was sometimes found in more than one dream from the same sleep session. One dream often connected with several childhood memories.

The similarity of cognitive content in the early memories and in the dreams was often accompanied by a similarity in the constellation of feelings implied by the cognitive content. In other instances, the feelings that were inherent in the dream content were different from the feelings implied in the early memory, although the cognitive content was similar. Themes that appeared in both memory and dream, and in the pattern of similarities and differences between them, also represented important personal characteristics of the individual.

The following example illustrates the similarity of cognitive content and of feeling constellation in earliest memory and dream. After the subincision film, one subject dreamed that he

> was at a lecture . . . it was like on an open campus and during . . . the speech . . . there were two planes flying by and one went into flames and crashed and . . . as it crashed I yelled "hit the dirt" and whoever was giving the speech said . . . "will you please leave." And I pointed to the crash and told him "look" and he saw it and bowed his head for a minute and that's when the phone rang.

In answer to the question about his earliest childhood recollections, during the interview conducted 9 months after this sleep session, the subject said:

> I remember about . . . the war mostly. When we used to have air raids. And turn the lights off and pull the shades down. People used to go around yelling, "Got your lights on. I'll break your windows." The air raid wardens, or what the story was.

These air raid drills also occurred in school. In another dream from the same sleep session, the subject dreamed that he had a case of "temporary blindness."

This subject said that he had watched the subincision film with "wonder" and "interest." The lecture setting for his dream and the classroom setting of his earliest memory are remarkably similar, and both reflect some detachment. This subject is a field-independent person. The cognitive content of both the airplane dream and the earliest memory contains the themes of danger from airplanes, of pulling shades down, and of people threatening. A similar constellation of feelings and ideas is reflected in the content of both the airplane and the "blindness" dreams and in the earliest memory. A prominent feature of the airplane dream and the earliest memory is the theme of a threatening and unjust authority, a theme readily evoked by the initiation rites in the subincision film. By implication, the subject's feeling is of resentment and in the airplane dream he is vindicated. There is other evidence in this subject's record of his open feelings of resentment and vindication.

Another example of similarity in both cognitive content and feeling constellation in dream and early memory comes from another subject, who dreamed, after the birth film, that at first he was in a nightclub, feeling nervous. Then he went to the bathroom. Then the scene changed and he was doing "calisthenics . . . all sorts of calisthenics. Situps, not situps, deep knee bends, running in place." One of this subject's early memories, offered spontaneously during the biographical interview some 8 months after the sleep session, was that "he didn't enjoy school at any time . . . I may have enjoyed one or two teachers, but otherwise I didn't enjoy school, at all. And I enjoyed the calisthenics." In this instance, the implied feeling carried by the reference to calisthenics in both the early memory and the dream is a feeling of relief of nervousness. This subject is a generally fearful person, and a field-dependent person.

In the next example, there is a cognitive link between the earliest memory and a dream, but the feelings implied are different. This subject dreamed after the subincision film that he

> was on the outskirts of a native village and I was supposed to be going someplace with the chief . . . and my daughter was following me and I was chasing her home . . . I had something in my hand uh it looks like one of these old-fashioned scoops that you scoop up . . . anything you bought loose, and it was made of rubber. It was flopping around in my hand. And I was taking a swipe or two at my daughter telling her to go home.

Asked about the scoop, he said it was what "grocers used to scoop up loose foodstuffs they used to keep in the drawers." As one of his earliest recollections, this subject said that

> when you hadda go down to the store or something these shadows would flicker across the halls. You'd run down like a shot and come up like a shot . . . and we had the neighborhood grocer . . . right downstairs.

The ideas of the "grocer," of "going someplace" one is "supposed to," and of "running" and "home" are contained in the earliest recollection and in the dream; the idea of the grocer's store and scoop makes a clear cognitive link. But the feelings implied in the earliest recollection and in the dream are different. In the dream, he is righteously indignant at his daughter for following him someplace where she does not belong. The feelings in the earliest recollection are of a frightened child, dutifully running between home and the grocer's store. The grocer's scoop, now flopping in the dreamer's hand, may be interpreted as condensed reference to present castration anxiety and past fright. This is also a field-independent person.

In the next example, a dream is connected to several earliest childhood recollections. The subject, reporting a dream after the subincision film, said that "one segment [of the dream] ironically dealt with the fact that I walked with my grandmother into a pet shop and wound up buying a rooster." His grandmother insisted on buying a smart-looking multicolored thing . . . and they bagged it like they would bag a dead chicken . . . We finally got this thing in the bag and we waited a few minutes and he was out of the bag and as he was about to be put back in the bag again the phone rang.

One of this subject's earliest recollections is placed when he was in an orphanage, and his "father came and saw me once and brought me a toy, like a monkey on a string that would go around." A nun took the toy away from him. The idea that connects the earliest recollection and the dream is that of the pet animal. Also similar is the idea of the older woman taking or wanting the toy. There is no actual identity of words, however, such as there was in the previous examples. In another of the subject's earliest recollections, his father again came to visit him and brought him "chicken," which he remembers he couldn't eat. The "dead chicken" idea in the dream is the same as the idea of chicken in this memory. The subject also remembers that his grandmother used to "feel the chickens" as she shopped in the market for the best one. The inference of a connection between earliest memories and the dream is strengthened by the single dream's connection to two different recollections of father's visits, and to the recollection of his grandmother going to market.

In the dream, the dreamer is amused at his grandmother's insistence on buying a pet cock, a clear double entendre for the penis. In general, this subject's recollections, though full of pathos, are good-humored and forgiving. His other dreams also have a considerable element of humor. This is a field-independent subject.

In the following example, a considerable amount of inference is needed to connect the cognitive content of the earliest recollection with the content of a dream. The inference, however, is in the nature of a symbolic translation of the dream content. The feeling states that characterize both the dream and the earliest recollection are almost identical.

The subject dreamed after the birth film that he was

riding on the subway . . . and a lady was selling raisin bread. And the subway wasn't moving. But . . . the lady had some kind of . . . some new kind of bread. But I didn't see no raisins . . . The bread had no crust . . . And this lady with a cart, selling raisin bread.

This subject's earliest recollection is as follows:

I don't know how old I was but I remember . . . I seen a woman nursing. And I guess I was old enough because she chased me away 'cause I was standing and watching her. I didn't know what she was doing. I never seen it before. She told me to go away.

The similarity in feeling state, especially in the stillness of things as he watched in his memory and in his dream, is striking. If we translate "raisin bread" as a breast symbol, there is also a similarity in cognitive content, including the "new kind" of bread, and the "nursing" he had never seen before. It is interesting that a characteristic theme of this dreamer's recollections is the theme of childhood innocence, now lost. The subject's first response to the request for biographical information was to volunteer that he was an illegitimate child. He was still not sure of the identity of his real mother.

The content of early memories also connects, in some instance, with dreams that occurred after the showing of neutral films. For example, the subject who dreamed about his grandmother and the rooster also dreamed, after the showing of the London film, that there was a baby "lying fully clothed in a crib . . . just toying . . . playing with his finger on the mattress." Here there is a similarity between the "toy" his father once brought him and "toying." Another of this subject's earliest recollections, this one specifically connected by him with his mother, is of having measles when he was 2 years old.

> In those days they used to take the children and have them completely nude in bed. Today, of course, it's a little different. The children wear pajamas and the window shades are down . . . I think my mother had me at someone's else's home.

This subject had formed the expectation that the experimenter was going to show him a sexually exciting film. He kidded the experimenter for thinking that the London travelogue could get him excited. Both his dream and his early recollection involve the theme of denial of sexual arousal. Inappropriate sexual activity is also a covert theme of his dream about his grandmother in the pet shop.

Another of this subject's early childhood memories is of having his head shaved when he was in the orphanage. He remembers also that when he was sent home, he was teased about his shaven head and called "curly." This recollection is an aid in interpreting the fact that this subject had an idiosyncratic autonomic arousal (respiration irregularity) during a portion of the subincision film when most subjects are relatively calm, that is, during a hair-tying scene that occurs in the middle of the film, after several scenes of penis incision. It is interesting, furthermore, that this subject had a very good-humored dream about the operator of a beauty salon (a thinly disguised reference to the experimenter) during the sleep session that included the far west travelogue, that is, a week after the subincision film was shown.

A review of these examples of the connections between early memories and dreams shows us an understandable route by which dream transformations of emotionally stirring events can occur. The person's affective responses to an event tap a cognitive structure (of emotionally congruent events) by which feelings are ordinarily encoded. This cognitive structure is embodied in images, words, and themes that, although personally idiosyncratic, understandably represent it. Once the person's unique allusions are known, we can trace the specific connections between the present stirring event and its coded version. Coding occurs by many different means: "gestalt" representation, associative linkage, coded "scenes." The person's cognitive style is also a factor in predicting characteristic feeling constellations and methods of both encoding and managing painful affects.

CHAPTER 4

Three Essays on the Theory of Sexuality
The Problem of Sex as Instinct

Freud's *Three Essays on the Theory of Sexuality* (1905), *Interpretation of Dreams* (1900), and *Studies on Hysteria* (Breuer & Freud, 1893–1895) are publications in which he set down his discovery that forbidden sexual longings were somehow transformed into neurotic symptoms. Although Freud's theorizing in *Three Essays* emphasized the primacy of instincts, the outcome of this work has been to focus attention on the primacy of human emotional—specifically, affectional-social—bonds as governors of human behavior.

As discussed in Volume 1, Freud could have focused his discovery of the emotional basis of mental illness on shame and guilt, the quintessentially social affective-cognitive states that involve both gross and subtle emotional exchanges between people. Instead, Freud focused on the sexual instinct (and its opponents) as the prime energetic sources of both symptoms and of the normal development of acculturated human beings. In his focus on sexuality, however, Freud, without explicitly saying so, was calling attention to the social nature of human nature. Partly as a result of his work, anthropologists now recognize that human culture, resting as it does on a long, intensely social infancy, is our species's unique evolutionary adaptation. I have suggested that culture involves people in the complicated states of shame and guilt from birth to death (Lewis, 1976), making them uniquely moral creatures.

In *Three Essays* Freud speaks of the "subordination" of sexual instinct to the "reproductive function" as "altruistic" (p. 207). Freud (1914) also calls attention to the social function of sex, saying that sex is unlike hunger and thirst because no one individual ever dies for lack of sex but the species would. In this sense, also, sex serves a social function. The impact of Freud's work on our understanding of the relationship between sex and social behavior went much further than these banal statements. The many lines of research into sexual behavior that have been inspired by Freud's formulations in *Three Essays* have amply demonstrated the wisdom of Freud's guess that sexuality reflects the prevailing social relationships in any culture, and that an individual's social relationships are heavily dependent on his or her psychosexual development. (The very term "psychosexual" is an outgrowth of Freud's thinking.) As a result of the questions that Freud raised in *Three Essays* we now understand that human evolution has been paralleled by the "socialization of sex" and by the "sexualization of society" (Beach, 1978, p. 19).

Studies of the nature of sexual behavior in primates and other non-human mammals have led to the understanding that sexual behavior is rooted in a matrix of social relationships. For example, the sexual capacity of adult mammals is strongly governed by their early social experiences (Harlow & Mears, 1979). In schematizing the mammalian mating sequence, summarizing many studies of animal sexual behavior (undertaken in response to Freud's work), Beach (1978) puts it this way: "Sexual activity is fundamentally a relational process, demanding interaction between two individuals" (p. 301).

In *Three Essays* Freud put forward his fundamental hypothesis that faulty sexual development has a negative effect on ego development. In fact, the outcome of the many studies growing out of this hypothesis has been strong evidence that the linkage is correct, but the statement is better turned upside down: Faulty ego development, that is, social development, has a negative effect on sexual behavior. So, for example, Money (1965) summarizes studies of both animal and human sexual aberrations as follows: "Any impedance of normal development and maturation, however seemingly remote from psychosexual identity, may have a noxious side-effect of psychosexual differentiation" (p. 13).

Paradoxically, then, although Freud formulated his observations in terms of the workings of a sexual instinct (thus affirming the materialist basis of his thought), the main outcome of his work on sexuality has been to demonstrate its profound roots in human social interaction. At the same time, his work has also demonstrated the sexual roots of human cultural institutions. Specifically, Freud showed that the emotional exchanges that govern human sexuality are far more potent than any instinctual forces. We now know that the affective states of shame and guilt are at least as powerful inhibitors (and sometimes instigators) of human sexual function as any hormones. We know also that the rageful and humiliated feelings that are intrinsic in shame and guilt may sometimes transform human sexual functioning into perversions: what Stoller (1975) aptly calls the "erotic form of hatred." Perhaps even more important, as Reich (1971) has shown, the understanding of such human cultural institutions as fascism is impossible without some comprehension of the sadistic-sexual components in human behavior that are fostered by an exploitative society (Lewis, 1976).

The best way to comprehend the scope of the questions Freud raised about sexuality (and his own uncertainty about theoretical formulations) is to review in detail the text of *Three Essays*. The editors of the *Standard Edition* tell us that Freud rewrote and revised *Three Essays* more often than any other publication save perhaps *The Interpretation of Dreams*. Although the editors do not say so, most of the revisions concern theoretical questions rather than changes in clinical observations, which have clearly stood the test of time.

ESSAY 1: ON PERVERSIONS

The main point of Essay 1, on the perversions, is Freud's discovery that neurotic symptoms

> give expression (by conversion) to [sexual] instincts which would be described as perverse in the widest sense if they could be expressed directly in phantasy and action without being diverted from consciousness. Thus, symptoms are formed at the cost of abnormal sexuality; *neuroses are, so to say, the negative of the perversions.* (p. 165, Freud's italics)

This discovery, in turn, involved a related one: that the adult perversions are not symptoms of degeneracy but are present in rudimentary form in the sexual life of children. The disposition of perversions thus "is no great rarity but must form a part of what passes as the normal constitution" (p. 171). Included in this normal constitution, already visible in childhood, are "component parts" of the sexual instinct that express themselves in all areas of the body—the mouth, anus, and skin—and somehow inhere in looking and touching, and in sadism and masochism. Freud observed a developmental series in which he could "trace the play of influences which will govern the evolution of infantile sexuality till its outcome in perversion, neurosis or normal sexual life" (p. 162).

By the "play of influences" Freud meant the interchange of emotions between the child and its caretaker around expressing "component instincts." But it remained for later psychoanalysts to spell out the affects involved. Klein (1948), for example, without altering Freud's theory of eros and the death instinct, spelled out the feelings of hatred, dread, loss and joy that characterize exchanges around "orality." Erikson (1950) transformed Freud's psychosexual instinct stages into corresponding affective-cognitive states—basic trust for satisfied orality, for example—thus converting Freud's instinct theory into an "object-relations" statement about "identity," but also without explicitly abandoning either instinct theory or libido theory.

Freud was clearly aware that *Three Essays* made "an attempt at enlarging the concept of sexuality" (p. 134). He also emphasized that this work was "deliberately independent of the findings of biology" (p. 131). But in order to deal with the "psychical manifestations of sexual life" (p. 217), Freud found it necessary to introduce hypothesis that sexual life has a special chemical basis for which he coined the term "libido." As discussed in Volume 1 (especially Chapter 3), in later writings Freud reluctantly abandoned his libido theory and, with it, a focus on a line of theorizing that could have posited the emotions as a central motivating force in human existence.

1. The Libido Concept

Freud had the genius to anticipate, in his concept of "libido," the existence of hormones as a special chemistry of sex. The subsequent discovery of hormones and their biochemistry has brought with it a growing understanding of the part they play not only in regulating sexual function but in somehow regulating the quality of emotional life. The gentling effects of estrogen and prolactin on the mothering behavior of mammals and the increase in aggressivity that comes with increases in circulating androgens are only two, now familiar, examples. If it were possible to telescope Freud's libido concept with present-day information, one might easily consider libido to be the psychophysiological construct underlying emotional life. It is fascinating that at least in one place in later writings, Freud actually wrote that "libido is an expression taken from the theory of emotions" (1921, p. 90).

Freud opens the first essay with a theoretical difficulty expressed semantically: He comments that language possesses no word to express sexual need in the way that "hunger" identifies nutritional needs. He offers the Latin word "libido" as a "scientific" way of describing sexual appetite, rejecting the (German) word *Lust*. In English as in German, *Lust* means, ambiguously, need (or tension) *and* gratification, two different experiences that Freud means to keep sharply differentiated. Freud's expressed reason for choosing "libido" over *Lust* is the ambiguity of the latter term with respect to tension or pleasure.

One can readily see how, by using a specially coined scientific term, Freud overcame not only the difficulty that *Lust* means both pleasure and tension, but also the difficulty that *Lust* also has a moral or ethical connotation. The conflict between desire and its opponents, guilt and shame, is clearly contained in the everyday usage of the term "lust." *Cassell's German-English Dictionary* lists "lascivious" and "lewd" as meanings of the German word; *Webster's English Dictionary* also tells us that "lust" has the meaning of "sinful desire" or "degrading passion." At the time *Three Essays* was published (1905b) Freud was much more interested in calling attention to the role of sexuality in human behavior than in describing the "counterforces." In *Three Essays* these are simply called "disgust," "shame," or "morality."

Freud's theoretical difficulties are actually rooted in this early choice of a "scientific" word for sexuality. Once having conceptualized neurosis in terms of the sexual instinct gone awry, Freud had endless trouble conceptualizing (as distinct from describing) the forces that inhibit or transform sex. Freud repeatedly described instances of the fact that human beings are fundamentally social, that is to say, moral-emotional creatures. But in the absence of a science of anthropology, he was unable to conceptualize the uniquely cultural basis of human nature, although he adumbrated it in *Totem and Taboo* (1913).

Freud was, of course, well aware of the theoretical difficulties in conceptualizing disgust, shame, and morality in terms of instincts. His way of dealing with the problem was to regard the counterforces as

> historical precipitates of the external inhibitions to which the sexual instinct has been subjected during the psychogenesis of the human race. We can observe the way in which, in the development of individuals, they arise at the appropriate moment, as though spontaneously, when upbringing and external influence give the signal. (p. 162)

In other words, Freud accepted the counterforces of shame, disgust, and morality as biological givens, along with sexuality. But he could not locate them, as we now can do, in the long-lasting affectional attachment system that is our species's unique form of adaptation.

In 1915 Freud added the section on "libido theory" to his *Three Essays*. This section, like his 1914 paper on narcissism, unequivocally stated the individualistic concept of human nature from which he then had to derive all the powerful effects of emotional conflict on sexual and

neurotic behavior that he had observed. The narrowness of the theoretical base that Freud constructed for himself is clearly apparent in this
section. He first defines libido as a "quantitatively variable force which
could serve as a measure of processes and transformations occurring in
the field of sexual excitation" (p. 217). He then delineates the "mental
representation" of the libido, to which he gives the name "ego-libido . . . whose production, increase or diminution, distribution and
displacement should afford us possibilities for explaining the psychosexual phenomena observed" (p. 217). But ego-libido is

> only conveniently accessible to analytic study when it has been put to the use
> of cathecting sexual objects, that is, when it has become object-libido . . . .
> We can follow the object-libido through still further vicissitudes. When it is
> withdrawn from objects, it is held in suspension in peculiar conditions of
> tension and is finally drawn back into the ego, so that it becomes ego-libido
> once again. In contrast to object-libido, we also describe ego-libido as "nar-
> cissistic" libido. . . . Narcissistic or ego-libido seems to be the great reservoir
> from which the object cathexes are sent out and into which they are with-
> drawn once more; the narcissistic libidinal cathexis of the ego is the original
> state of things, realized in earliest childhood and merely covered by the later
> extrusions of libido, but in essentials persists behind them. (pp. 217–218)

The obvious theoretical obscurities in this section (as well as in the
1914 paper on narcissism) have been one source of experimentalists'
derision for Freud. It is of course unclear how one can use a concept of
ego-libido that is by definition inaccessible to observation until it has
changed into object-libido. Even more important, "object relations"
must, in this theoretical framework, be derived from ego-libido or narcissistic libido. For Freud, emotional relationships between infant and
caretaker are thus secondary outgrowths of primary narcissism. This is a
theoretical stance that our newer knowledge of infancy calls into question (e.g., Ainsworth, 1979; Bowlby, 1969; Hogan, 1975; M. Lewis &
Brooks-Gunn, 1979).

Freud was forced to rely on the then prevailing instinct theory to
account for both sexuality and morality, although he himself clearly
recognized its limitations in failing to take sufficient account of learning
and emotional experience. In his paper *On Narcissism* (1914), Freud laments the "total absence of any theory of instincts that would help us to
find our bearings" (p. 78). But some form of instinct theory was necessary for a scientist in the Darwinian era; otherwise one might have to
rely on the theologian-philosophers. In addition, Freud's attention was
caught by the characteristic of the sexual experience that arousal, although pleasurable, is also tension producing (that is, unpleasurable),
whereas orgasm (also pleasurable) is tension releasing, resembling the
pattern of discharge of nerve impulse with which Freud was so familiar

as a neurologist. It was at this level of conceptualization that he formulated his unique contribution to instinct theory: the libido as a special chemistry of sex.

The perspective of this level of conceptualization is that of the individual organism in the sense that it focuses on the ebb and flow of intrapsychic forces. These are, however, readily responsive to stimuli in the environment, including other persons. In a footnote, the editors of the *Standard Edition* (p. 217) call attention to the ambiguity of Freud's use of the term "libido" when he describes libido as "concentrating on objects." They remind the reader that Freud means "concentrating on mental presentations of objects and not, of course, objects in the external world." We are thus reminded of the confusion inherent in switching between levels of conceptualization, and inherent in not allowing the psychological level its own place in nature. At the physiological level, which is the place of the libido concept, individual organs and organ systems are being studied; at the psychological level, when sexual longing or arousal is involved, it is the interaction between the person and his or her physical and social surround that is studied. Novikoff (1945) has helped to clarify a concept of hierarchies of conceptualization in nature with the following statement:

> Each level of organization possesses unique properties of structure and behavior which, though dependent on the properties of the constituent elements, appear only when those elements are combined into a new system. (p. 209)

In *Three Essays* we find Freud attempting to make the libido concept explain the complicated social phenomena that instinct theory could not otherwise comprehend. The libido concept is an attempt to encompass the psychophysiology of sexual emotions. When, in addition, Freud later (1926) abandoned his libido theory of neurosis in favor of a biological stance, the marriage between Freudian psychoanalysis and "primary narcissism" was sealed. In short, the heart of *Three Essays*, which is Freud's inspired idea that human emotional relatedness governs both neurotic and normal behavior, has been obscured by the book's theoretical framework, as happened also in *The Interpretation of Dreams*.

2. Comparisons of Primate and Human Sexuality: Social versus Hormonal (Libidinal) Control

As we shall see in Chapter 8, the "scientific myth" (as he himself called it) that Freud developed to account for the genesis of guilt (*Totem and Taboo*, 1913) sketched a pattern of primate or early human behavior in terms of family dynamics or emotional interactions culminating in patricide. Comparisons of primate and human sexual regulation have since become a major concern of experimental psychologists (and they are still struggling, as Freud was, not only with tendencies to anthropomorphize animal behavior, but also with the biases that inhere in automatically equating human and nonhuman aggression).

We now know from the work of some anthropologists and experimental psychologists (e.g., Ford & Beach, 1951) that the outstanding difference between primate and human sexual regulation is in the extent of hormonal control: Human sexuality is comparatively free of hormonal (libidinal) control. It is thus ironic that Freud's attempt to rescue "libido" from the pejorative meaning of *Lust* is much more applicable to nonhuman species' sexuality, in which hormones do play a more decisive role than in ourselves. In primate social groups, in which mating can occur only when the female is in estrus, the males' orderly access to the female is "arranged" by contest between individual males. The acquisition of "dominance" status is, however, not simply a question of brute strength but of social skills as well. "No monkey becomes dominant merely on the basis of fighting skill, nor is dominance a permanent property of an individual" (Bernstein, 1978, p. 153). Freud's concept of a dominant "father-male" keeping the juvenile males in submission by brute strength was biased in its emphasis on the role of aggression in primate groups.

To explain mating behavior in higher mammals, Darwin (1871) had invoked two main selective agencies, combat or competition (usually between males) and preference by females for certain characteristics of their mates. In subsequent years, evolutionists placed major stress on male size and aggressiveness as the prime "natural selection" factor. (This emphasis on brute strength in the male is an example of the androcentric attitude then and still prevalent in science.[1] What this emphasis ignored was the implication that selection operates against the smaller, less aggressive female (Bernstein, 1978). No species can long survive that selects against females. Workers in the field of primate biology are still debating the genetic mechanisms involved in sexual selection. Freud's insight, however, that human sexual selection is unique in being governed by morality has been amply confirmed, if only in anthropologists' finding of a worldwide incest taboo.

Another consequence of the loss of estrus with its clock-signal for sexual arousal is the circumstance that human sexuality is not seasonal

---

[1]For a fuller discussion of sexism in evolutionary theory see my *Psychic War in Men and Women*. (Lewis, 1976).

but continuous. It is also unique in its responsiveness to social institutions both as stimulus and as inhibitor of sexual arousal. One way of describing this unique human condition is to say that human sexuality is under more cortical than hormonal control (Beach, 1978; Ford & Beach, 1951). Still another phrasing, which owes much to Freud, suggests that the estrus stimulus has been replaced by profound emotions of mutual commitment and love. Primate biologists point out that the affectionate and social behaviors that adult nonhumans show in abundance have little, if anything, to do with primate copulation. But primate-type affectionate and social behaviors, such as kissing, grooming and high-spirited playfulness have been incorporated into the human sex act (usually when two people are making love, not just copulating).

In *Three Essays* Freud clearly enunciated the close linkage between affectional and sensual currents of behavior. "Should the two currents fail to converge, the result is often that one of the ideals of sexual life, the focusing of all desire upon a single object, will be unattainable" (p. 200). Freud followed up this observation with evidence from psychoanalytic cases in which failure of the two currents to unite resulted in psychical impotence in men (Freud, 1910). (In this 1910 publication he clearly described the affectionate current as the "older of the two," p. 180.) When, at puberty, the sensual current seeks only an incestuous figure, the male may be impotent except with persons he devalues or debases.

Even more important, Freud clearly predicted that disturbances in the "affectionate currents" during childhood can seriously impede adult sexuality. Speaking of maternal love, Freud wrote: "What we call affection will unfailingly show its effects one day on the genitals as well" (p. 223). This prediction has been amply confirmed in the work of the Harlows. Harlow and Mears (1979), for example, start with the premise that the behavior of both primates and human beings is founded on "the various forms of love and affection," with human motives being only more "subtle and persistent" than those of primates (p. 8). They find that the "so-called primary drives of hunger, fear, rage and pain are actually socially disruptive" and not a proper basis for explaining the behavior of social animals such as monkeys and human beings (p. 8). Using a "human model" of affectionate mother–infant interchange in infancy as their guide, Harlow and Mears summarize an enormous number of studies that observe the devastating effects of maternal deprivation on adult sexuality. To have anticipated such major findings is a tribute to Freud's genius in observing the connection between early affectionate interaction and adult sexuality.[2] Freud's theoretical concept,

---

[2]It is remarkable that Harlow and Mears's volume contains no reference to Freud.

however, in spite of many revisions by him, still failed to take account of the affectionate and social nature of the human beast.

3. Freud's Critique of the Sexual Instinct

While proposing a new concept, libido, to account for the energy of the sexual instinct, Freud simultaneously undertook a critique of the conventional notion that heterosexuality is simply instinctive, and of the correlative notion that homosexuality is likewise innate. Carefully distinguishing between the *object* of the instinct and the *aim* of the instinct (Freud's italics), the latter being the "act toward which the instinct tends" (p. 136), Freud observed that there can be many variations in the object or person sought, as well as in sexual aim. The main point of Freud's critique of the sexual instinct was to emphasize the role of learning and early experience in governing the choice of both object and aim. His emphasis on the role of learning and individual experience and on the useless antithesis between innate and acquired stimuli should gladden the heart of the most orthodox present-day behaviorist.

Freud's critique of the sexual instinct was so thoroughgoing that, at a time when he was also combating the "scientific" view that sexual deviations reflect human "degeneracy," he also opened up the question of how heterosexual choice comes about. He wrote:

> Thus, from the point of view of psychoanalysis the exclusive sexual interest felt by women for men is also a problem (along with inversion) that needs elucidating and is not a self-evident fact based upon an attraction that is ultimately of a chemical nature. (p. 146)

Beach (1978, p. 2), writing nearly three-quarters of a century later, still tells us that the "etiology of exclusive heterosexuality is far from perfectly understood."

Examining Freud's careful distinction between object and aim makes it clear that he actually had enormous difficulty in keeping the concept of aim distinguished from its object. The careful distinction turns out to reflect much less of a difference than appears at first sight because the "object," that is, the person involved, is so overwhelming a determinant of aim.

The category of aim appears to contain two subcategories: first, the sexual act, and second, the tension discharge accompanying it. In the first category Freud contrasts genital with nongenital aims. Freud observed that the aim of the adult sexual act need not be copulation, but might involve nongenital activity—"certain intermediate relations to the sexual object such as touching and looking at it" (p. 149), or kissing in which parts of the body not directly genital are involved. What Freud overlooks is that these intermediate sexual acts or nongenital aims have clear reference to a variety of sexual objects, all of which have the symbolic significance of another person. In fact, in his discussion of deviations with respect to aim Freud is in the contradictory position of citing the "overevaluation of the sexual object" as an instance of deviated aim (p. 150)! Freud himself is aware of the contradiction. In discussing fetishism he writes:

> From the point of view of classification, we should no doubt have done better to have mentioned this highly interesting group of aberrations of the sexual instinct among the deviations in respect to sexual *object* (Freud's italics). But we have postponed their mention until we could become acquainted with the factor of sexual overevaluation, on which these phenomena, being connected with an abandonment of the sexual aim, are dependent. (p. 153)

This explanation seems quite obscure, since overevaluation is about "objects" or persons as well as involving the aim of including the "object's" whole body (not just the genitals) in the sexual act. Thus it is apparent that the social interactions implicit in the sexual act were the phenomena on which Freud was focusing in his critique of the sexual instinct.

Homosexuality. Freud adduced a number of observations about homosexuality that speak against the sexual instinct as an explanatory concept. He observed, first of all, that inverts form a "connected series" (p. 138), ranging from persons who can have orgasm only with a same-sex partner to persons who are only occasionally homosexual. The connected series varies also along a continuum of homosexuals' attitudes about inversion, from homosexuals who are troubled to those who are relatively accepting of their inversion. Freud's observations were not systematically pursued until the Kinsey studies (Kinsey, Pomeroy, & Martin, 1948; Kinsey, Pomeroy, Martin, & Gebhard, 1953). (It is remarkable that a cross-sectional study of American sexuality was undertaken not by a psychologist, or a sociologist, but by someone whose original training was as an entomologist.) Kinsey's studies confirmed Freud's notion that homosexuals form a "connected series." Those studies also adduced powerful evidence that sexual practices vary with age, socioeconomic status, religious beliefs, and with sex, thus reflecting the influence of experiential factors. Anthropologists' catalogs of the multiplicity of norms governing human sexual behavior are even more overwhelming evidence of its essentially social nature (see, e.g., Davenport, 1978).

Freud also insisted that the "mental quality of masculinity" is often found among male homosexuals. He thus carefully separated masculine and feminine personality from sexual object-choice as well as from innate sex. Freud's distinction is one that present-day psychologists phrase as the difference between "gender role" and sexual choice. With hindsight it is clear that attention to Freud's observation could have prevented the tortuous course that afflicted the study of masculinity and femininity, especially in American psychology. As Constantinople (1973) has decisively shown in her literature review, for many years tests of masculinity–femininity erroneously assumed that it is unidimensional in nature. This erroneous assumption rested, in turn, on the assumption that "normal" males inevitably (both by nature and nurture) show masculine traits and females feminine ones, so that the frequency of a trait among males and females could be used as a measure of masculinity and femininity. Present-day work on psychological androgyny is an outgrowth of our corrected view of masculinity and femininity. Freud, however, was unmistakably clear in his observation that masculine and feminine personality does not coincide either with sex or with sexual choice.

As one example of the continuing usefulness of Freud's distinction between heterosexuality and masculinity–femininity, an empirical study (Storms, 1980) has recently shown that sexual orientation is more closely related to the character of erotic fantasies than it is to masculinity–femininity (as measured by Spence-Helmreich). Storms asked college students of both sexes to label themselves "gay," "straight," or "bisexual." These labels proved not to be related to their masculinity–femininity scores; they were, however, congruent with the androcentric or gynoerotic content of their erotic fantasies. Storms suggests that his results strongly support the Freudian view that people are inherently bisexual, that is, equally capable of responding sexually to either gender.

Freud also observed in *Three Essays* that homosexuals need not be otherwise disturbed personalities. In fact, Freud had concluded that homosexuals are people whose "efficiency is unimpaired and who are indeed distinguished by a specially high intellectual development and ethical culture" (p. 139). Freud's accepting attitude toward homosexuals foreshadowed the 1952 deletion of homosexuality as a category of pathology from the American Psychiatric Association's diagnostic manual, a deletion that continues, despite controversy, to the present day. Ironically, although many psychoanalysts are opposed to the deletion, it could not have taken place without Freud's insight that homosexuality does not necessarily involve pathological personality.

Sexual Perversions.   Freud's view was that there is little or no relationship between personality and other adult sexual deviations, such as child molesting or intercourse with animals. As he understood it, disturbances in adult personality and social relationships (neurosis) were invariably linked with (unconscious) deviations in sexuality. But the converse—that adult sexual deviants are *always* otherwise disturbed people—was not true. He wrote:

> In my experience anyone who is in any way, whether socially or ethically, abnormal mentally is invariably abnormal also in his sexual life. But many people are abnormal in their sexual life, who in every other respect approximate to the average, and have, along with the rest, passed through the process of human cultural development, in which sexuality remains the weak spot. (p. 149)

Freud reiterated this view after his discussion of all the sexual perversions, including the most repulsive.

> Here again we cannot escape from the fact that people whose behavior is in other respects normal can, under the domination of the most unruly of all the instincts, put themselves in the category of sick persons in the single sphere of sexual life. On the other hand, manifest abnormality in the other relations of life can invariably be shown to have a background of abnormal sexual conduct. (p. 161)

His interpretation of the absence of necessary connection between overt perversion and other personal abnormality was that

> the mental factor must be regarded as playing its largest part in the transformation of the sexual instinct. It is impossible to deny that in their case [perverts] a piece of mental work has been performed which, in spite of its horrifying result, is the equivalent of an idealization of the instinct. The omnipotence of love is perhaps never more strongly proved than in such aberrations as these. The highest and lowest are always close to each other in the sphere of sexuality: "von Himmel durch die Welt zur Hölle." (pp. 161–162)

His observation that sexual perversions can exist in an otherwise "approximately" normal person and his interpretation of this phenomenon as the result of a "transformation"—that is, a "piece of mental work . . . the equivalent of an *idealization of an instinct*" (p. 161, italics added)—is an instance in which Freud implicitly relies on the social nature of human nature. Recognition of the primacy of human emotional relatedness makes the most horrible perversions—licking excrement or having intercourse with dead bodies—more comprehensible. Freud calls these examples extreme cases in which the "sexual instinct goes to astonishing lengths in successfully overcoming the resistances of shame, disgust, horror or pain" (p. 161). The term "idealization of an instinct" itself implies the primacy of emotional and social attitudes toward the instinct. In fact, Freud relied on the idealization of the sexual instinct to explain the difference between our civilization and that of antiquity. In a much quoted footnote, he wrote:

> The most striking differentiation between the erotic life of antiquity and our own no doubt lies in the fact that the ancients laid stress upon the instinct itself, whereas we emphasize its object. The ancients glorified the instinct and were prepared on its account to honour even an inferior object; while we despise the instinctual activity in itself, and find excuses for it only in the merits of the object. (p. 149)

Freud's wistful reference to a time when sexual longing was presumably less troubled by the forces of shame and guilt, less requiring of "excuses," is apparent in that footnote. He was, moreover, using the term "instinct" to represent behavior profoundly governed by the broader circumstances of social and emotional life.

In conceptualizing the "component instincts" or "erotogenic zones," however, Freud tied them to the narrowest physiological base of the instinct concept: "The source of an instinct is a process of excitation occurring in an organ and the immediate aim of the instinct lies in the removal of this organic stimulus" (p. 168). The editors of the *Standard Edition* point out that this sentence appeared only in later editions of *Three Essays*; in earlier editions, Freud had conceptualized the component instincts as including motor impulses that are nonsexual. Even this change reflects Freud's difficulty in deciding on his theoretical terms. And even "motor impulses," like sexual ones, move the organism toward or away from other persons or things. Libidinal tension and discharge, in contrast, are intrapsychic processes. In summary, then, Freud's observations about the social nature of even the most repulsive perversions were lost in his theoretical formulations about the nature of instincts.

ESSAY 2: INFANTILE SEXUALITY

1. Infantile Amnesia

It is noteworthy that a discussion of infantile amnesia precedes Freud's discussion of infantile sexuality. Freud emphasizes that loss of memory for childhood events is a product of repression, that is, of the counterforces of guilt and shame. Once again, he clearly places infantile sexuality in a context of emotional and social relatedness.

Freud opens his essay on infantile sexuality by expressing his astonishment that scholars have written so extensively about primeval or hereditary sexuality, but have studiously avoided describing the sexual life of children. In a 1910 footnote he tells us that he checked this "bold" assertion by doing a review of the literature of the intervening 5 years and found the situation essentially unaltered. He attributes this strange neglect not only to "considerations of propriety" on the part of scholars, but to the "astonishing" existence of infantile amnesia, a phenomenon not yet understood, but of the utmost importance for the understanding both of hysteria and of normal functioning. Freud regards the phenomenon of infantile amnesia as all the more astonishing because there is strong evidence (from other people's accounts of our behavior) that as children

> we reacted in a lively manner to impressions, that we were capable of expressing pain and joy in a human fashion, that we gave evidence of love, jealousy and other passionate feelings by which we were strongly moved at the time, and even that we gave utterance to remarks which were regarded by adults as good evidence of our possessing insight and the beginnings of a capacity for judgment. And of all of this we, when we are grown up, have no knowledge of our own! (pp. 174–175)

Freud attributes at least some instances of infantile amnesia to the repression of shameful and guilt-inducing events, basing this observation upon his own self-analysis.

In an earlier paper on screen memories (1899), Freud had written a thinly disguised autobiographical account of one of his own earliest memories. In that paper he raised fascinating questions about the functioning of memory in general. He suggested, for example, the existence of cognitive-affective schemata, within which seemingly meaningless memory fragments become intelligible. In this line of reasoning he clearly anticipated the modern-day concept of "scripts" (Abelson, 1981) governing recall. Reflecting on the origin of conscious memories in general, Freud separated emotionally governed screen memories from ordinary recollections. These latter phenomena could be explained by the "simple view that they arise simultaneously with an experience and thereafter they recur . . . according to the familiar laws of reproduction." He then rejected this simple view, observing that in the majority of recollections the subject

> sees himself in the recollection as a child, with the knowledge that this child is himself; he sees this child, however, as an observer from outside the scene would see him. . . . Now it is evident that such a picture cannot be an exact repetition of the impression that was originally received. For the subject was then in the middle of the situation and not attending to himself but to the external world. (1899, p. 321)

In this passage Freud is making use of a concept of the self, contrasting the participating with the observing self. As a result of this distinction he is led to question whether we ever have memories *of* childhood, suggesting instead that our memories may be *related to* childhood (Freud's italics), forming themselves out of experience as it touches the self. The capacity of infantile amnesia to abolish our recollections of infantile sexual experiences is thus a function of the moral schemata in which development takes place.

2. The Latency Period: Morality Building

The sexual life of children is not only subject to amnesia, but it is normally "overtaken by a progressive process of suppression" (p. 176). In describing the interaction between infantile sexuality and its restraints, Freud writes: "There seems no doubt that the germs of sexual impulses are already present in the newborn child and that these continue to develop for a time" (p. 176).

That the germs of sexual impulse are present in newborn children was, in fact, an inspired guess, since we now know that penile erections are regularly recurring events during the REM cycle of newborns. The erections are part of a syndrome of REM cycle "arousal," but they are also neonate forerunners of cyclically recurring penile erections during the normal REM sleep of adults.

Freud also distinguishes a "period of partial or total latency" during which there are "built up the mental forces which are later to impede the course of sexual instinct and, like dams, restrict its flow—disgust, feelings of shame and the claims of aesthetic and moral ideals" (p. 176). As we have already seen, the dam-building process of morality is itself instinctive. In fact, the "moral defensive forces" are themselves constructed "at the cost of sexuality" (p. 179).

It should be noted, also, that Freud is very tentative about the process of morality building. He makes the suggestion, first, that the sexual impulses of childhood cannot be utilized since the reproduction function is deferred. For this reason, they are diverted from their sexual aims to social ones by the process of "sublimation." Second, the sexual impulses are perverse, arising from erotogenic zones, and "because they go contrary to the direction of the subject's development, can only arouse unpleasurable feelings" (p. 178). In order to suppress these unpleasurable feelings, sexual impulses evoke opposing mental forces that build up the dams of disgust, shame, and morality. Freud is referring in this second process to the mechanism he termed "reaction formation," in which the instinctual energy is used for the suppression of specific sexual impulses, rather than being more generally diverted from sexual aims.

In these observations Freud has all the ingredients of a social theory of human nature: a uniquely human morality based on the maintenance of affectional (sexual) bonds. But his formulations in terms of tension building and discharge (libido) took him in the direction of a narcissistic theory of human nature.

3. Manifestations of Infantile Sexuality

Thumb Sucking. Freud chooses, as his first and best example of infantile sexuality, the appearance of thumb sucking early in infancy. "Sensual sucking," as he calls it, is not the same as sucking for nutritive purposes, but involves grasping another part of the infant's body and some rhythmical activities. The fact that pediatricians and other observers of infancy do not regard thumb sucking as sexual is ascribed by Freud to a confusion between "sexual" and "genital." After a thorough discussion of thumb sucking, he offers to give the criteria for regarding it as sexual, criteria that turn out to be more question-begging than convincing.

Let us first follow Freud in his descriptive examination of thumb sucking. He tells us:

> The most striking feature of this sexual activity is that the instinct is not directed toward other people but obtains satisfaction for the subject's own body. It is "autoerotic", by a happily chosen term introduced by Havelock Ellis. (p. 181)

Having just stated that thumb sucking is *not* directed toward other people but is autoerotic, Freud proceeds immediately to say that "it is determined by a search for some pleasure which has already been experienced and is now remembered. . . . [The child] is striving to renew" the pleasures experienced at the mother's breast. The child's lips "behave like an erotogenic zone and no doubt stimulation by the warm flow of milk is the cause of the pleasurable sensation" (p. 181).

Freud's theoretical formulation of the relationship between the pleasures of thumb sucking and the pleasures of nutritive sucking is that they represent two separate instinctual currents—sex and hunger. This notion is based on an individualistic concept of human nature. It concentrates on the intrapsychic ebb and flow of pleasure and tension. The evidence for the concept of an infant as a social organism by biological endowment (e.g., Rheingold, 1969) was simply not available to Freud.

Freud's assumption of an individualistic concept of human nature is further emphasized by a sentence added to *Three Essays* in 1915 (after his 1914 paper on narcissism): "To begin with, sexual activity attaches itself to functions serving the purpose of self-preservation and does not become independent of them until after" (p. 182). "Self-preservation," in other words, is the primary force in human nature; sexual activity begins in the service of self-preservation. As we shall see later in this chapter, this formulation is partly the result of a confusion between a concept of "self" and a concept of the "ego." If the ego is used to denote the whole organism, then "self-preservation," or more accurately, "ego-preservation" is primary. This is, however, as Freud often recognized, a tautology. But if ego is distinguished from the self, with the latter having the meaning of our uniquely human capacity for judging ourselves in our own and others' eyes, then sexual activity need not be conceptualized as inherently ego preserving. Even the most egotistical forms that sexual activity takes can be shown to be self-preservative—that is, defensive of threatened affectional bonds. Sexual activity is inherently social (like the rest of our functioning), even when it is antisocial. This is the paradox that Durkheim and G. H. Mead, as well as Freud, have helped us to understand.

Freud concludes his description of thumb sucking or sensual sucking by offering the promised set of criteria for calling it sexual. The first is that it attaches itself to a vital somatic function, such as eating; the second is that it has *no* sexual *object;* and the third is that its sexual *aim* is dominated by an erotogenic zone. These three criteria, however, are hardly indicative of the sexuality of thumb sucking, since the first two are nonsexual and the third simply describes the pleasure of both nutritive and nonnutritive sucking. All three criteria, however, can fit the concept of a bonding or emotional attachment between infant and mother, for which thumb sucking becomes a (pleasurable) signal.

It should be noted that Freud is puzzled by his own formulation: He wonders why "in order to remove one stimulus, it seems necessary to adduce a second one at the same spot" (p. 185). The focus of Freud's puzzlement centers on the mechanism by which the need for a repetition of the satisfaction arises.

> The state of being in need of a repetition of the satisfaction reveals itself in two ways: by a peculiar feeling of tensions, possessing, rather the character of unpleasure, and by a sensation of itching or stimulation which is *centrally conditioned and projected on to the erotogenic peripheral zone* [italics added]. We can therefore reformulate a sexual aim in another way: It consists of replacing the projected sensation of stimulation in the erotogenic zone by an *external stimulus* [italics added] which removes the sensation by producing a feeling of satisfaction. This external stimulation will usually consist of some kind of manipulation that is analogous to the sucking. (p. 184)

As we follow the tortuous line of reasoning about how a second stimulus occurs at the "same spot" as the first need, it is clear that Freud's problem would have been simplified by the adoption of the idea that there is satisfaction inherent in the infant–mother relationship. Substitutes for the relationship and signals of it can themselves become satisfying in the ever-widening growth of the infant's experience.

Masturbation. Freud used thumb sucking as his model for other autoerotic activities, including masturbation. In the model, all zones of the body are inherently capable, like the lips, of becoming erotogenic zones. In the case of the anal zone, the involvement of somatic functioning is clear, as it is in the case of the genitalia. Freud describes the pleasure of both anal excretion and anal retention in clearly social terms. The feces are the child's first " 'gift'; by producing them he can express his active compliance with the environment, by withholding them, disobedience" (p. 186). The anatomical closeness between the genitalia and the anus and urinary tracts involves the latter in masturbatory gratifications, so that the foundations for later genital primacy are established early in infancy.

In discussing the "oscillations" of infantile sexuality, Freud attaches *"great and lasting importance . . .* to *accidental contingencies"* (p. 190, Freud's italics). He does not retract his observation that seduction by adults is a significant factor in the etiology of hysteria, conceding only that he "overrated" its importance compared to intrinsic infantile sexuality. (As the editors of the *Standard Edition* remark, p. 128, Freud blows hot and cold on the issue of adult seduction of children.) When describing the seduction of children Freud is very sensitive to the emotional-social situation that seduction represents:

> Seduction . . . treats the child as a sexual object prematurely and teaches him in highly emotional circumstances how to obtain gratification from his genital zone, a satisfaction he is obliged to repeat again and again by masturbation. (p. 190)

But the lesson Freud learns from this is that children are instinctively polymorphously perverse! They can be "led into all possible kinds of sexual irregularities" (p. 190) because of this inherent sexuality.

To emphasize children's polymorphous perversity, Freud, in one of his misogynist pronouncements, proceeds to compare children to the

> average uncultivated woman in whom the same polymorphous perverse disposition persists. Under ordinary conditions she may remain normal sexually, but if she is led on by a clever seducer she will find every sort of perversion to her taste, and will retain them as part of her own sexual activities. Prostitutes exploit the same polymorphous, that is, infantile, disposition for the purposes of their profession; and, considering the immense number of women who are prostitutes or who must be supposed to have an

aptitude for prostitution without becoming engaged in it, it becomes impossible not to recognize that this same fundamental disposition to perversions of every kind is a general and fundamental human characteristic. (p. 191)

We are reminded here sharply of the way in which Freud's individualistic formulation of the sexual instinct makes him miss the very social and emotional forces that he is himself describing. This is the same contradiction that led him to formulate Dora's dilemma in terms of her unruly sexuality rather than in terms of a personal betrayal by both Herr K. and her father (see Volume 1, Chapter 3).

Scopophilia, Exhibitionism, and Sadism. The contradiction in Freud's theorizing about sexuality is highlighted by the difficulties he encountered in conceptualizing his observations about scopophilia, exhibitionism, and sadism. For example, he attributed curiosity—our "instinct of knowledge"—to a "sublimation that makes use of the energy of scopophilia."

> The threat to the bases of a child's existence offered by the discovery or the suspicion of the arrival of a new baby and the fear that he may, as a result of it, cease to be cared for and loved, make him thoughtful and clear-sighted. (pp. 194–195)

Freud observes, moreover, that the child's frustrations in his attempts to understand such significant emotional events in his life as childbirth, sexual intercourse, and mother's pregnancy may lead to a "high degree of alienation of the child from the people in his environment who formerly enjoyed his complete confidence" (p. 197). Once again, Freud is embedding intellectual activity in the child's ongoing affectional bonds. But, theoretically, intellectual activity is a sublimated "narcissistic" love of looking at the self!

Scopophilia, exhibitionism, and sadism are components that do not directly relate to parts of the body. Therefore, Freud writes, "It must be admitted . . . that infantile sexual life, in spite of the preponderating dominance of erotogenic zones, exhibits components which *from the very first involve other people as sexual objects*" (pp. 191–192, italics added). Scopophilia, exhibitionism, and sadism are indeed easier to conceptualize if they are regarded as products of attachment.

When conceptualizing thumb sucking, anal-erotism, and masturbation, Freud had been able to point to a zone of the body, or to the whole surface and interior of the body, as the somatic source of the instinct. But sexual pleasure when looking at other people's genitals or having one's own looked at, and sexual pleasure in effecting or contemplating other people's suffering cannot be related to body stimulation alone. In *Three Essays* Freud makes an attempt to keep the body connection by treating looking as some kind of substitute for touching, and by supposing that pleasure in cruelty has something to do with the experience of mastery. But the emotional relationship between the self of the voyeur or the sadist and the self of someone else is so obvious that it cannot be denied. The emotional states of triumph and humiliation, in which the self participates vicariously in the loved person's humiliation (shame) or triumph, could not, however, be conceptualized by Freud as products of attachment.

The issue of conceptualizing attachment as a "given" is at the basis of Freud's discussion in his later metapsychological papers of the vexing question whether "object-libido" should be kept separate from "ego-libido," or whether it should be subsumed, as it was by Jung, under one all-purpose heading of "psychic energy." The term "object-libido" was Freud's substitute for sexual libido and always clearly referred to loving other people, or their symbolic substitutes. He therefore clung to it as a hallmark of psychoanalysis. When it came to ego-libido, particularly in the absence of a concept of a socially formed self, Freud felt obliged to postulate that libido actually inhered in the ego but was observable only when it attached itself to "objects."

The difficulties Freud encountered in his theorizing are apparent in the very questions he asked himself. For example, asking what makes it necessary for a theory to go beyond narcissism (or ego-libido), he answers with a reference to the necessity for loving others: "A strong egoism is a protection against falling ill, but in the last resort we must begin to love in order not to fall ill, and we are bound to fall ill if, in consequence of frustration, we are unable to love" (1914, p. 85). Freud's theoretical underpinning for the conception, however, is that the ego cannot take an excessive amount of stimulation and so must direct libido outward: "our mental apparatus is first and foremost a device for mastering excitation which would otherwise be felt as distressing or would have pathogenic effects" (ibid.).

As we have already seen, a related problem that created difficulties for Freud was the conceptual distinction between the "ego" and the "self." This distinction is one that has since caught the attention not only of such psychoanalysts as Sullivan and Binswanger, but of many psychologists as well (e.g., Allport, 1943; Chein, 1944; Lewis, 1958). The concept of the self as an organizing, experiential system into which the "other" is inextricably woven from earliest infancy was simply not available to Freud. Freud used the term "ego" sometimes to refer to the self with this implicit meaning and at other times to a "mental apparatus for mastering excitation" (1914, p. 85).

Freud made frequent clinical use of the concept of the self. In his paper on narcissism (1914), for example, he offers some remarks on the subject of "self-regard." He distinguishes between normal and neurotic self-regard. The latter derives from the fact that loving is repressed rather than "ego-syntonic." When repressed, loving someone else involves such a "severe depletion of the ego" that replenishment requires a return to "narcissism [which] represents, as it were, a happy love" (1914, p. 100). When one is in love "neurotically" there is so much shame or humiliation involved (vis-à-vis the other) that narcissism is invoked as a balm to the "depleted" self.

Once again the outlines of an attachment theory of human nature are visible. But without a concept of the self as a product of earliest and ongoing social-emotional interactions, the phenomena of scopophilia, exhibitionism, and sadism–masochism must be dealt with as regressions to narcissism, instead of modes of interaction in the struggle to maintain affectional ties.

In his theoretical papers on metapsychology, Freud clearly describes the vicariousness or social connectedness inherent in the "instinctual impulses" of sadism–masochism and exhibitionism–scopophilia. For example, he writes: "Analytic observation . . . leaves us in no doubt that the masochist *shares in the enjoyment of the assault upon himself,* and that *the exhibitionist shares in the enjoyment* of the [sight of] his exposure" (1915a, p. 127, italics added). (Freud's demonstration of the interchangeability of the "object" and "subject" in sadism–masochism and scopophilia–exhibitionism prompted the editors of the *Standard Edition* to comment in a footnote that there is some "confusion." Although the editors do not say so, we can assume that the confusion is inherent in vicarious experience.)

But in theorizing about the origins of sadism and scopophilia without the benefit of a concept of the (social) self, Freud of necessity looked to the bodily organ in which these "instincts" should have their narcissistic source. Clearly, however, the "object" of scopophilia is not the eye itself, nor is the musculature the "object" of sadism. Freud therefore had to hedge about his notion that the origin of these partial instincts is in the body, and he supposed that there must be an "object other than itself" (p. 132) involved.

Perhaps the clearest evidence for the difficulty Freud had in fitting emotions into his theoretical scheme of things emerges when one reads his discussion of love and hate. He writes (1915a, p. 133):

> The case of love and hate acquires a special interest from the circumstance that *it refuses to be fitted into our scheme of the instincts* [italics added]. It is impossible to doubt that there is the most intimate relation between these two opposite feelings and sexual life, but we are naturally unwilling to think

of love as being some kind of special component instinct of sexuality in the same way as the others we have been discussing. We should prefer to regard loving as the expression of the *whole* current of feeling (Freud's italics); but this idea does not clear up our difficulties, and we cannot see what meaning attaches to an opposite content of this current [i.e., hate].

Freud's attempted solution is to postulate that

> at the very beginning of mental life [there is the] condition "narcissism". . . . At this time the external world is not cathected with interest (in a general sense) and is indifferent for purposes of satisfaction. During this period, therefore, the ego-subject coincides with what is pleasurable and the external world with what is indifferent (or possibly unpleasurable), as being a source of stimulation. (1915a, pp. 134–135)

As we follow his attempted solution it is clear that the "external world" to which Freud is referring is not the mothering person. (Once again, the editors here call attention to difficulties in understanding Freud's "condensed" writings.) Freud develops an explanation of the transformations of love into hate that relies on the connection between "pleasure" and loving and the parallel connection between "unpleasure" and hating. In this respect, he is making use of a rudimentary conditioning theory. Freud also finds it necessary to distinguish between the "pleasure-ego" and the "reality-ego," the latter being the infant's biologically given awareness of needs that cannot be satisfied "from within." Even with these props, the theoretical system is in difficulties that Freud himself recognizes:

> We might say at a pinch of an instinct that it "loves" the object towards which it strives for purposes of satisfaction; but to say that an instinct "hates" an object strikes us as odd. Thus we become aware that *the attitudes of love and hate cannot be made use of for the relations of instincts to their objects but are reserved for the relations of the total ego to objects.* (1915a, p. 137, italics added)

It seems likely that Freud's "total ego" is a reference to the self as an organizing system of experience, and that a positive relationship between the self and the other is a necessary concept for the understanding of both love and hate. In any case, the clinical phenomena of sadism–masochism and of scopophilia–exhibitionism that encompass such exquisite mixtures of love and hate are very difficult to encompass in a theoretical system that has no concept of a social self.

Developmental Psychosexual Phases. Freud's theoretical conception of the developmental phases—oral, anal, and phallic—was also very different from his clinical description of them as affective experiences. For example, the more theoretical section on the phases (added to *Three Essays* in 1915) speaks of the oral state as "cannibalistic." In the same paragraph, however, the sexual aim of the oral stage is called "incorporation of the object," and this incorporation is called "the prototype of a process . . . of identification" (1905b, p. 198). "Identification" and "incorporation" are very different concepts; yet the latter can be understood as a metaphor for the former. In identification, the vicarious experience of the other person's affect is the means by which self takes the other's place, metaphorically incorporating the other. Describing the infant as "cannibalistic," in contrast, refers to Freud's theory that human beings are intrinsically "narcissistic." This was the line of theorizing that would ultimately lead Freud to his concept of a death instinct.

The Sources of Infantile Sexuality. In the final section of Essay 2, Freud discusses the origin of the sexual instinct. He reviews his description of the erotogenic zones of the body and of the musculature as sources of sexual excitement. Freud also emphasizes that "all comparatively intense affective processes, including even terrifying ones, trench upon sexuality" (p. 203). Freud's clinical description vividly portrays how the frightened or angry child may be sexually aroused. By Freudian inference, moreover, the sexual arousal may be understood as a symbolic summoning of the significant other person to the rescue of the child's self.

It is instructive, also, to realize that the sexually arousing properties of emotional arousal are currently being studied. A recent experiment (Wolchik, Beggs, Wincze, Sakheim, Barlow, & Mavissakalian, 1980) demonstrated that viewing emotionally arousing films had significant effects on men's sexual arousal as measured by a penile strain gauge. The experimenters themselves make no mention of Freud, referring instead to Wolpe.

ESSAY 3: THE TRANSFORMATIONS OF PUBERTY

In tracing the changes that puberty brings to infantile sexual life, thus finally shaping adult sexuality, Freud pinpoints three major problems. These are the change from predominantly autoerotic to "object" love; the subordination of the erotogenic zones to genital primacy; and the differentiation between men and women. Freud uses a simile to describe the formation of adult sexuality:

> It is like the completion of a tunnel which has been driven through a hill from both directions. . . . The main requirement of adulthood is that there be an exact convergence of the affectionate and the sensual current, both being directed toward the sexual object and the sexual aim. (p. 207)

In discussing the problem of genital primacy, Freud's attention is caught by the probability of an underlying sexual chemistry, that is, by the libido theory. In discussing the problem of object love, Freud leans heavily on a social theory of sexual development. The contrast between these two levels of conceptualization is very sharp in the essay on adult sexuality. The difficulties that Freud encountered as a result are no-where more apparent than in his treatment of the differentiation be-tween the sexes. Freud had clearly kept concepts of masculinity and femininity separate from sexual behavior or sex role in Essay 1. But in Essay 3, his views on masculinity and femininity can be interpreted as a compromise between social and "libidinal" influences, with the latter predominant, so that social influences are only vaguely mentioned. Since Freud devoted only two pages of Essay 3 to the differentiation between the sexes, and since the controversy he engendered was and still is far-reaching, we shall postpone a full discussion of his views on this subject to the next chapter.

1. Genital Primacy and Forepleasure

The problem Freud poses is understanding the psychology of "sexual excitement." He describes two sorts of "indications" of the experience of sexual excitement, "mental" and "somatic." The mental indicators he describes as a "peculiar feeling of tension of an extremely compelling character" (p. 108), whereas the somatic indicators are an obvious preparation for the sexual act—"the erection of the male organ and the lubrication of the vagina" (p. 208). It is the mental indicator—tension—that puzzles Freud because (as we saw in Essay 1) tension is both pleasurable and unpleasurable. "How, then, are this unpleasurable tension and this feeling of pleasure to be reconciled?" (p. 209).

Freud laments as the "sore spot" in psychology that so little is known about pleasure and unpleasure (a lament that is almost as apt in 1983 as it was in 1905). In trying to solve this puzzle, Freud turns his attention to the way in which the erotogenic zones fit into the new arrangements at puberty. Their existence accounts for the state of mounting excitement in which "an experience of pleasure can give rise to a need for greater pleasure" (p. 210). The need for greater pleasure leads to an increase in tension which in turn produces "the necessary motor energy for the conclusion of the sexual act" (ibid.). This last act (orgasm) is wholly pleasurable and is not accompanied by further in-crease of tension; in fact, it is accompanied by discharge of tension. Freud coined the terms "forepleasure" for the mounting-excitement phase and "end-pleasure" for orgasm. It is forepleasure that is clearly connected with infantile sexual life, whereas end-pleasure is something new that comes with puberty.

The formula for the *new function* [italics added] of the erotogenic zones [is that] they are used to make possible, through the medium of the fore-pleasure which can be derived from them (as it was during infantile life) the production of the greater pleasure of full satisfaction. (p. 211)

This formula, however, does not really account at all for why mounting tension (or unpleasure) should accompany mounting pleasure. Freud makes no use of his own insight that each of the erotogenic zones that can be involved in forepleasure is symbolic of complicated (and ambivalent) emotional interactions with significant other people. One source of tension along with pleasure can be the simultaneous activation of inhibitory signals derived from the "forepleasure" or erotogenic zones.

Freud does, in fact, hint at this aspect of things in a footnote in which he reminds the reader that the "forepleasure" found in joking is "used to liberate a greater pleasure derived from the removal of internal inhibitions" (p. 211). This is an insight that Freud documented fully in his book on jokes (1905a). In Essay 3, however, Freud's attention is devoted to the striking characteristic of tension that it seems to reflect the operation of sexual chemistry. Although he discounts an explanation of tension that ties it only to the accumulation of semen (this model being indadequate to account for the phenomenon in women and in children), he is clearly drawn to special chemistry. He even suggests that neuroses show the greatest "clinical similarity to the phenomena of intoxication and abstinence" (p. 216). How easy it is to bypass emotional interactions when "toxic" substances can be invoked.

2. Finding an Object

In describing adult object-finding, Freud makes his famous statement: "The finding of an object is in fact a re-finding of it" (p. 222). In a footnote, Freud makes the distinction between "anaclitic" and "narcissistic" modes of object-finding in infancy. He makes the point that narcissistic attachment is of great importance only in pathological cases, whereas normal development involves social attachment. He seems to imply that social relationships are primary sources of sexual love when he writes: "A child's intercourse with anyone responsible for his care affords him an unending source of sexual excitement and satisfaction from his erotogenic zones" (p. 223).

In discussing the incest barrier, Freud relies on a social explanation for its existence: "Respect for this barrier is essentially a cultural demand made by society" (p. 225). The repudiation of the inevitable incestuous

fantasies that arise in the life of each person is "one of the most significant, but also one of the most painful, psychical achievements" of
puberty. It accomplishes the necessary "detachment from parental authority, a progress that alone makes possible the opposition, which is so
important for the progress of civilization, between the new generation
and the old" (p. 227).

In the same paragraph in which Freud tells us that some people
(neurotics) are unable to get over their parents' authority, he also tells us
that the most vulnerable are "girls, who to the delight of their parents,
have persisted in their childish love far beyond puberty" (p. 227). Once
again, however, the social conditions that might underlie such vulnerability are bypassed in favor of an explanation that relies on an "infantile fixation of the libido."

Let us now recapitulate the many lines of inquiry that Freud opened
up in *Three Essays*. The relationship between social and sexual development has been demonstrated in a wide range of studies of the mother–infant interaction among both primates and humans. The existence
of hormones regulating emotional life, including sexual feeling and behavior, was foreshadowed by Freud's libido concept. The fact that homosexuality and other deviations form a connected series with "normalcy" is another of Freud's important observations, based on his
recognition of the potency of social interactions in sexual life. His attitude of scientific inquiry into the perversions has itself been a major
factor in changing sexual mores. Even more important, Freud's inquiry
into the concept of "normalcy" called into question conventional beliefs.

Freud's discovery of the sexual currents in infants' and children's
lives is another of his inspired guesses. Our present-day information
that cyclically recurring penile erections during REM sleep occur in infancy emphasizes Freuds discovery. Perhaps the most important consequence of *Three Essays*, however, is that it gave clear expression to the
idea that human emotional relatedness, of which sex is so central a part,
governs both neurotic and normal behavior.

CHAPTER 5

Anatomy is Destiny
The Problem of Freud's Sexism

In many ways, Freud's views on the personality differences implicit in being a man or a woman illuminate the political basis and the political implications of psychological views on human nature. To the extent that Freud saw human nature as sexually repressed by civilization, his work tended toward the liberation of both sexes from their culturally stereotyped sex roles. However, he embedded his clinical observations about sexual repression and resulting neurosis in a scientific framework of instinct theory. The instinct theory that he devised, though progressive in the sense that it was materialist, could also be used as an implicit justification for domination, specifically for domination by men over women. These issues are still being hotly debated today in discussions of social Darwinism (see, e.g., Tobach & Rosoff, 1978).

Freud believed that he was describing different patterns of (sexual) attachment and development in the two sexes. If the inevitable consequence of the differing patterns was women's constitutional inferiority, that was lamentable, but it was a fact of life. For these views he is regarded by many feminists as an enemy of women's liberation. Within academic psychology also, opposition to Freud's biologism is voiced by social learning theory (Mischel, 1966), by leading students of cognitive-developmental theory (Kohlberg, 1966), and in the empirical work on sex differences (Maccoby & Jacklin, 1974). As we shall see in this chapter, however, Freud's idea that experience with early caretakers is different for the two sexes has been a powerful stimulus to the development of new information about how the two sexes grow, and even to new programs for the social reform of the family, such as "parenting" (Dinnerstein, 1977; Chodorow, 1978; Baumrind, 1980). Freudian—that is, primary-process—interpretations of the personality differences inherent in being a woman or a man continue to provide us with insights, in spite of Freud's sexism.

SEXISM: A FREUDIAN CONCEPT

With the revival of the feminist movement in recent years, Freud has been sharply criticized, and justly, as a sexist. Misogynist statements in Freud's writings are not hard to find. As one example, we have seen his likening the polymorphous perversity of children to the sexual behavior of women. Here is another, even more damaging, example: In his paper on narcissism (1914) Freud writes that

> complete object-love of the attachment type . . . is characteristic of the male. Women are by nature more subject to an intensification of their original narcissism. Strictly speaking, it is only themselves that women love. (p. 89)

And, according to Freud, this narcissism is what gives women (also children and criminals) their special charm!

There is no question, also, that Freud was subject to the androcentric attitudes of his time—attitudes that are still very potent today. Freud often lamented his own inability to understand women's psychology. So, for example, in a 1923 postscript to *Three Essays* Freud explicitly tells us that he can describe the infantile genital organization of the libido "only as it affects the male child; the corresponding processes in little girls are not known to us" (p. 142).

The very concept, however, of a "sexist," or of sexist thinking, and the specific distortions that accompany androcentrism and misogyny, are insights that we owe to Freud's rich description of emotional defenses. It is now generally recognized, even among some orthodox psychoanalysts (e.g., Chassaguet-Smirgel, 1970), that Freud was unwittingly rationalizing women's social inferiority when he treated the absence of a penis as an actual constitutional defect.

Theodora Wells's (personal communication) script revising Freud's ideas about anatomy and destiny illustrates the irony that Freud's mistakes can best be illuminated by Freud's own methods of interpreting (some) mistakes as primary-process thinking—in this instance, accomplishing the aggrandizement of males. The script contains Wells's account of how psychoanalysis might sound if women were in positions of power. It is designed as an introduction to therapy sessions for distressed, inferior males.

> Feel into the fact that women are the leaders, the power centers, the prime movers. Man, whose natural role is husband and father, fulfills himself through nurturing children and making the home a refuge for the woman. This is only natural to balance the biological role of woman who devotes her whole body to the race during pregnancy: the most revered power known to Woman (and to men, of course). Then feel further into the obvious biological explanation for woman as the ideal: her genital construction. By design, female genitals are compact and internal, protected by her body. Male genitals are exposed so that he must be protected from outside attack to assure the perpetuation of the race. His vulnerability obviously requires sheltering. Thus, by nature, males are more passive than females and have a desire in sexual relations to be symbolically engulfed by the protective body of women. Males psychologically yearn for this protection, fully realizing their masculinity at this time and feeling exposed and vulnerable at other times. A man experiences himself as a "whole man" when thus engulfed. If the male denies these feelings, he is unconsciously rejecting his masculinity. Therapy is thus indicated to help him adjust to his own nature. Of course, therapy is administered by a woman, who has the education and wisdom to facilitate openness leading to the male's growth and self-actualization. To help him feel into the defensive emotionality he is invited to get in touch with the child in him. He remembers his sisters' jeering at his primitive genitals that "flap around foolishly." She can run, climb and ride horseback unencumbered. Obviously, since she is free to move, she is encouraged to develop her body and mind in preparation for her active responsibilities of adult womanhood. The male vulnerability needs female protection so he is taught the less active, but caring virtues of homemaking.Because of his vagina-envy he learns to bind up his genitals and learns to feel ashamed because of his nocturnal emissions. Instead, he is encouraged to dream of getting married, waiting for the time of his fulfillment—when "his woman" gives him a girl-child to care for. He knows that if it is a boy-child he has failed somehow—but they can try again. In getting to the child in him these early experiences are reawakened. He is, of course, led by a woman and in a circle of nineteen men and four women as he begins to work through some of his deep feelings of inferiority.

My point is that this script could not have been written without Freud's methods of interpreting as primary-process what seems to be straightforward cognitive content.

Freud's discoveries were made in an intellectual tradition stemming from the Enlightenment, and indeed from classical antiquity (e.g., in the epic of Lucretius, *De Rerum Natura*)—a tradition that detailed the baleful effects of human civilization on human beings. One thread of that tradition held that civilization itself is inimical to humanity. Rousseau, for example, described how civilized human beings had lost their compassion (*pitie*). Another element of the tradition denied any intrinsic opposition between society and the individual, but rather saw an exploitative society as destructive of human nature; thus Marx emphasized the alienation of spirit that capitalism breeds, and more recently the Marxist Freudians—notably Wilhelm Reich and Erich Fromm—have traced in detail how an exploitative society deforms human relatedness. Feminist social criticism is still another legacy of the Enlightenment. And although feminist thinkers are divided about the noxious role of the profit system, they are united in directing their criticism against the personal deformations that result from the widespread social inferiority of women.

Freud's critique of civilization posited an inherent conflict between the individual and a social order built upon the painful repression of sexuality. Thus there is implicit in Freud's work a critique of the morality on which the social order is based. Once the morality of the social order is brought into question, social inequality, particularly the subjugation of women, cannot be comfortably accepted; it must be "rationalized"— something Freud was very skilled at doing himself as well as describing in others. In spite of Freud's misogyny and his androcentrism, however, his actual discovery of the power of human emotional bonds in the acculturation process has made it possible to investigate how the two sexes are differently acculturated in both exploitative and nonexploitative societies (Lewis, 1976). In particular, I have stressed the differential proneness of women and men to states of shame and guilt in the struggle to stay acculturated.

ANDROCENTRISM IN BIOLOGY: FREUD'S HERITAGE

As we saw in Chapter 4, evolutionary theory as Freud knew it emphasized male aggression, that is, skill and cunning in fighting, as the prime selection factor in human adaptation. Freud was also working in an atmosphere that took for granted that women, although childbearers, were the "second sex." One consequence is that Freudian instinct theory ignored the basic long-lasting affectional ties that make human beings cultural animals, at the same time that Freud was actually describing the powerful emotional forces, including sexual feelings, that govern human attachment behavior in the nuclear family.

The prevailing androcentrism in biology is well illustrated by the history of ethology, one of the recently developed methodologies that have significantly altered the climate of thinking in the behavioral sciences. Relying on the *de novo* observations that were the hallmark of the nineteenth-century naturalists, and in which the behavior observed was altered as little as possible by the observation itself, ethologists have called attention to the *social* conditions governing even the narrowest neurophysiological responses (Chance, 1980). Chance points out, for example, that Pavlov did not inquire into the extent to which his experimental dogs were social creatures. Recognizing the social character of the animal, however, makes an enormous difference to even so narrow a function as the salivary reflex. Denton (cited by Chance, 1980), for example, showed that although sheep ordinarily salivate constantly, the rate of salivation can be augmented naturally, not at the sight of food, but at the sight of another sheep feeding. When, therefore, food is brought to a solitary sheep in a laboratory, the salivary reflex is absent and no conditioning by the experimenter is possible. But if another sheep is brought in and fed in the laboratory, conditioning of the first sheep becomes possible.

Another consequence of the neglect of the social interactions governing behavior has been the failure to recognize that the adult animal's social relationships "assume equal if not greater importance than his direct relationship to the physical environment" (Chance, 1980, p. 87). Two distinct patterns of social attention have been discerned in nonhuman primates, namely, the agonic and the hedonic modes of social cohesion. In the agonic mode, which is originally based on responses to the threat of physical danger, the threat has been encapsulated within the group by the existence of a dominant male, who serves as a focus of social attention but is also a "negative social referent." In the hedonic mode, which also fosters group cohesion, other animals are "positive social referents," in the context of which eating, resting, sleeping, and grooming take place.

Chance points out that the existence of a separate hedonic mode of social interaction has been the "single most important discovery" resulting from ethologists' focus on patterns of social attention in primate groups.

> The integrity of the . . . hedonic system has been hidden as its components—involving body contact (as in grooming, sitting or sleeping next to), relaxation and exploration . . . appear at different times. . . . Only when the elimination of danger occurs, as within the core of a territory, or when the young are in the presence of the mother and in contact with her, has the hedonic system been seen as a single piece. (p. 89)

Chance suggests that the reason for the relatively late discovery of a hedonic mode was the fact that ethology developed initially from the study of birds and fishes, whose social relations are phasic and constructed on agonic forms. Another reason that seems equally plausible is the prevailing androcentrism in science, which regarded affectional bonds as secondary derivatives of individualistic instinct or drives. The mother–infant interaction was neglected both as a factor in the evolution of species (see Elaine Morgan's *The Descent of Woman*, 1973) and as a central "biological" source of humanity's long-lasting affectional and moral bonds. As we have already seen, Freud was also a captive of the prevailing androcentric attitudes.

Another very illuminating example of androcentrism in Freud's time comes from the history of embryology. In Freud's time (before the discovery of the chromosomal basis of sex), it was known that the reproductive system is undifferentiated in the very early fetal stages. The genital tubercle that forms in both sexes later becomes the clitoris in the female and the penis in the male. The generally accepted doctrine interpreted these facts as meaning that the clitoris is a vestigial or abbreviated penis; from which Freud speculated that by adulthood women should have outgrown the need for this vestigial organ, and for him this speculation somehow gained the status of a phylogenetic fact.

In relatively recent times, since the discovery of the chromosomal basis of sex and the hormones that chromosomes release, embryologists have discovered that without the operation of the y chromosome the embryo remains female. This leads to a concept of a model, or "template," of the embryo as basically female. Sherfey (1972) tells the story of how hard it was for embryologists in the 1940s (mostly men) to grasp this concept. She says that it was only when she read the statement that "the neuter sex is female" that she herself grasped that some primary-process thinking was in evidence. Scientists were having a hard time announcing to the world that the Adam's rib belonged to Eve.

Freud was aware of the extent of his own ignorance about women. He lamented it frequently, not only in the 1923 quotation cited earlier, but twice again in 1924 (Fliegel, 1973). At the same time (in a familiar Freudian mechanism called projection), he often cast the blame for his ignorance on the women themselves. Thus he writes that the erotic life of women "partly owing to the stunting effect of civilized conditions and partly owing to their conventional secretiveness and insincerity, is still veiled in impenetrable obscurity" (1905b, p. 151). Another example of Freud's prejudice against women is in his treatment of their sociability or moral development. He observed that the "development of the inhibitions against sexuality [shame, disgust, pity, etc.] takes place in girls earlier and in the face of less resistance than boys." But this does not mean to him—as it might have, in terms of his own system—that the moral development of girls is faster and less difficult than that of boys. Rather, in the very sentence just quoted he continues, "the tendency to sexual repression seems in general to be greater; and where the component instincts of sexuality appear, they prefer the passive form in girls" (1905b, p. 219). One does not need to be a very accomplished Freudian to recognize that the earlier and easier development of socialization in girls is being interpreted to their disadvantage as a function of their having a less active sexual instinct. As we shall see in this chapter, there is now strong experimental evidence that girls are more sociable than boys (Maccoby & Jacklin, 1974). Girls' aggressions are more "prosocial," that is, more "moral," than boys' (Sears, Rau, & Alpert, 1965)—still another confirmation of Freud's observations rather than of his theory. We shall return to this question of moral development in Chapter 8.

Freud's sexism is particularly visible in the open contradictions within his own model of psychosexual development for the two sexes. In one model in *Three Essays* (1905b), Freud assumes that women's development is homologous to men's, an attitude that considers women to be the "other sex" but otherwise implies the equality of the sexes. The oedipal triangle is homologous for the two sexes, based on a component of heterosexual attraction that is the same for both. The sexual fantasies of the two sexes are equally incestuous and "differentiated owing to the attraction of the opposite sex—the son being drawn toward his mother and the daughter toward her father" (p. 227).

Freud, however, had already contradicted his homologue version of the model of psychosexual development when he wrote, a few pages earlier in *Three Essays* (1905b), that "libido is invariably and necessarily of a masculine nature, whether it occurs in men or in women, and irrespectively of whether its object is a man or a woman" (p. 218). Because libido is masculine, the model of psychosexual development is male for both sexes; women's task in development is to repudiate their masculinity. This is, of course, the model that brought much criticism within the psychoanalytic movement, as we shall see in a moment when we examine the history of Horney's controversy with Freud. But it is the model to which Freud clung; he repeated it in his final publication on the subject of women: "We are now obliged to recognize that the little girl is a little man" (1933, p. 118).

Freud's model was thus one of equality when he was thinking about "the object relations" of the two sexes. It was when he was thinking of their genital zones that women could not be allowed to enjoy the clitoris. Freud apparently could not believe that the clitoris (even though it was a homologue of the penis) could be, or should be, a source of orgasm for the adult woman. The following somewhat extended quotation of a famous passage in his writings makes clear the operation of

Freud's sexist bias. He was thinking about women's sexuality from the man's point of view.

> If we are to understand how a little girl turns into a woman, we must follow the further vicissitudes of [this] excitability of the clitoris. Puberty, which brings about so great an accession of libido in boys, is marked in girls by a fresh wave of *repression* (Freud's italics) in which it is precisely clitoridal sexuality that is affected. What is thus overtaken by repression is a piece of masculine sexuality. *The intensification of the brake upon sexuality brought about by pubertal repression in women serves as a stimulus to the libido of men and causes an increase of its activity. Along with this heightening of libido there is also an increase of sexual overvaluation which only emerges in full force in relation to a woman who holds herself back and who denies her sexuality* [italics added). When at last the sexual act is permitted and the clitoris itself becomes excited, it still retains a function: the task, namely, of transmitting the excitation to the adjacent female sexual parts, just as—to use a simile—pine shavings can be kindled in order to set a log of harder wood on fire. . . . When erotogenic susceptibility to stimulation has been successfully transferred by a woman from the clitoris to the vaginal orifice, it implies that she has adopted a new leading zone for the purpose of her later sexual activity. A man, on the other hand, retains his leading zones unchanged from childhood. The fact that women change their leading erotogenic zones in this way, together with the wave of repression at puberty, which as it were, puts aside their childish masculinity, as the chief determinants of the greater proneness of women to neurosis and especially to hysteria. These determinants, therefore are intimately related to the essence of femininity. (p. 220)

It is amply clear from this passage that "femininity" is tailored to fit men's needs.

As Freud saw it, moreover, the assumption of their adult role was a harder task for women than for men. If one follows this line of reasoning, women should be more prone than men to disturbances of gender identity. We now know, in fact, that the reverse is true. Men are more prone than women to all disorders of gender identity (see Volume 1, Chapter 5). And although women are more prone than men to hysteria, they are not more prone to mental illness in general. Men are more prone not only to disorders of gender identity and sexual functioning, but to obsessional neurosis and paranoia. Freud (1909) himself suggested an affinity between obsessional neurosis and masculinity.

Freud's sexism is apparent not only in *Three Essays* but also in his 1918 paper on *The Taboo of Virginity* (where his misogyny is also very visible). Freud recognizes that the high value placed by civilized men on virginity is something needing explanation, instead of being taken for granted. His own explanation, however, goes no further than taking for granted the existence of (male-dominated) monogamy as a reflection of the development of civilization. Placing a high value on virginity, he says, is the "logical continuation of the right to exclusive possession of a woman which forms the essence of monogamy" (1918, p. 193).

How is it, then, that primitive peroples do not have the same regard for virginity that we do? Freud's interpretation is that the taboo of virginity is an instance of the generalized dread of women. "Perhaps this dread," he writes,

> is based on the fact that woman is different from man, forever incomprehensible and mysterious, strange and therefore apparently hostile. The man is afraid of being weakened by the woman, infected with her femininity, and of then showing himself incapable. The effect which coitus has of discharging tension and causing flaccidity may be the prototype of what the man fears; and the realization of the influence which the woman gains over him through sexual intercourse, the consideration she thereby forces from him, may justify the extension of his fear. In all this there is nothing obsolete, nothing which is still not alive among ourselves. (pp. 198–199)

At this point, Freud is being very Freudian—that is, interpreting primary-process ideation in which women might be experienced as irrationally frightening. But in the next moment, in the same paper, he is arguing that "danger *really exists* [italics added], so that with the taboo of virginity a primitive man is defending himself against a correctly sensed, although physical danger" (p. 201). (Once again, as was pointed out in Chapter 3 of Volume 1, Freud is ambiguous as to whether emotional danger is "real" or "physical.") The danger is that the woman's hostility will be evoked by her defloration "and the prospective husband is just the person who would have every reason to avoid such enmity" (p. 202). The woman's hostility, moreover, is evoked not by the pain of her defloration (and the invasion of her body) but by her penis envy!

> Behind this envy for the penis, there comes to light the woman's hostile bitterness against the man, which never completely disappears in the relations between the sexes, and is clearly indicated in the strivings and in the literary productions of 'emancipated' women. (p. 205)

Summing up, Freud writes:

> A woman's *immature sexuality* is discharged onto the man who first makes her acquainted with the sexual act. This being so, the taboo of virginity is reasonable enough and we can understand the rule which decrees that precisely the man who is to enter upon a life shared with this woman shall avoid these dangers. (p. 206)

As evidence for the survival of this wisdom he cites a popular comedy of the day entitled *Virgin's Venom*, which reminds him of the "habit of snake-charmers, who make poisonous snakes first bite a piece of cloth in order to handle them afterwards without danger" (p. 206). The imagery he uses in this instance suggests more than a touch of misogyny.

Freud's Misogyny: The Horney Story

There was, as already suggested, a streak of misogyny in Freud. At the time Freud was working androcentrism did not go unchallenged in all quarters. John Stuart Mill and Friedrich Engels were only two of the very influential, eloquent voices calling attention to the subjugation of women. Not only did Freud ignore these challenges to androcentrism, but, as we shall see in a moment, he dealt very harshly with critics within the psychoanalytic movement who questioned his views on the constitutional inferiority of women. In any case, even though Freud welcomed many women as his students, the combination of prevailing androcentrism and Freud's misogyny have made many of his clinical pronouncements on the sexuality of women demonstrably wrong, an unusual fate for Freud's clinical observations. For example, his dictum that it is necessary for women to overcome their liking for clitoral orgasm has been overturned by subsequent evidence (Masters & Johnson, 1970), but many women patients suffered considerable harm in the interim.

The history of the controversy between Freud and Karen Horney, a controversy that led ultimately to her defection from the Freudian movement and the development of her own school of psychoanalysis, has been carefully researched by Zenia Fliegel (1973). It is a story illustrating the fact that Freud did not use his own method of primary-process interpretation of the emotions engendered by sex. If he had, the sexism inherent in his own views might have been more clearly apparent to him—as it was to Horney.

By the time Horney came to write her paper on the genesis of the castration complex in women, in 1922, Adler had already been read out of the Freudian movement for suggesting that "feelings of inferiority" in a competitive world were a source of emotional conflict and neurosis. Adler had also suggested that women are prone to inferiority feelings in response to their actual subordination in society. Horney's 1922 paper was written within the Freudian psychoanalytic movement; it was read at the Seventh International Congress of Psychoanalysis in Berlin. Horney took issue with Abraham's and Freud's assumption

> as an axiomatic fact that females feel at a disadvantage because of their genital organs without this being regarded as constituting a problem in itself—possibly because to masculine narcissism this has seemed too self-evident to need explanation.

Horney goes on to say that

> an assertion that one half of the human race is discontented with the sex

assigned to it and can overcome this discontent only in favorable circumstances—is decidedly unsatisfying, not only to feminine narcissism but also
to biological science. (Horney, 1922/1967, p. 38)

As one reads this paper, it is clear that the suggestions she makes
rely heavily on the Freudian assumption that our ideas about the role of
men and women are primary-process transformations representing conflicted feelings. As Fliegel says, one can hardly escape the judgment that
Horney was more Freudian than Freud in grasping the importance of
infantile sexual *fantasies* about the anatomies, rather than clinging to a
notion that the absence of a penis actually makes women constitutionally inferior.

Horney makes three specific suggestions about why little girls respond enviously to the realization that boys have a penis. Each of
Horney's suggestions is a very Freudian interpretation based on clinical
material from her own cases. This evidence links penis envy to "urethral
erotism," "scopophilia," and "masturbation wishes." In explaining
urethral erotism, Horney suggests that children "narcissistically over-
value" all their excretory functions. Fantasies of omnipotence are more
easily associated with the "jet of urine" passed by the male. Horney
cites a frequent game played by two little boys in which they urinate to
make a cross which will kill the person they are thinking of at the
moment. As for scopophilia, little girls cannot see their genitals. "Woman can arrive at no clear knowledge about her person and therefore finds
it harder to free herself from herself" (Horney, 1922/1967, p. 41). As for
masturbation wishes, girls have a harder time overcoming these because
they sense that boys do gratify themselves every time they hold their
penis to urinate. It is apparent that each of these interpretations of early
penis envy is made within the spirit and even the letter of Freudian
thinking.

Horney's major point of disagreement with Freud is voiced along
with a grateful acknowledgment of how much Freud's paper on homosexuality in women helped her to understand the castration complex in
women (p. 49). The point of disagreement is that, according to Horney,
women's neurotic attitudes toward the penis are not based on their early
or primary penis envy, but also on later disappointments and experiences of humiliation in their oedipal attachment to their fathers. Horney's view of the decisive importance of the later disappointments of
women is based on her own clinical observations. She writes:

> The numerous unmistakable observations . . . show us how important it is
> to realize that . . . as an ontogenetic repetition of a phylogentic experience

the child constructs, on the basis of a (hostile or loving) identification with its mother, a fantasy that it has suffered full sexual appropriation by the father; and further, that in fantasy this experience presents itself as having actually taken place—as much a fact as it must have been at that distant time when all women were primarily the property of the father. (p. 44)

Horney thus attributed the castration complex in neurotic women to the reactivation of their early penis envy as a consequence of disturbed object relations. Evidence from her own cases had persuaded her that women's castration complex was a defense against guilty fantasies of rape and castration at the hands of their fathers. She suggested, moreover, that healthy women do get over their early penis envy through a positive identification with their mothers, including a wish to be like them in having a child by a man. So far, as we read the text of her 1922 paper, there seems little to evoke controversy within the psychoanalytic movement. On the contrary, one might have thought that Horney's clinical observations would be welcomed as useful additional information about the development of women, especially since Freud had so often acknowledged his own ignorance of the psychology of women.

Horney's paper met a very different fate. Freud pointedly ignored it, except for a passing reference to it in his famous paper on the anatomical distinction between the sexes (1925). In that paper he behaved as if there were no differences between her views and his own, but for the first time he laid down an authoritative description of girls' psychosexual development, and from then on he never revised it. As Fliegel (1973) observes, reading Freud's paper after reading Horney's suggests that Freud's "formulations constitute a direct reversal" (p. 389) of Horney's thesis. In Freud's formulation, a girl's oedipal wishes develop only out of frustrated phallic jealousy and out of forced resignation to her actually castrated condition.

Fliegel's hypothesis to account for Freud's sudden adoption of an authoritative position on the subject of women was that he had developed cancer in the interval between Horney's 1922 paper and his 1925 publication. Freud's introduction to his paper is indeed explicit in his reference to a shortened life span. He also clearly suggests that he is publishing without waiting for confirmation of his views, a practice that he reminds his readers is not his custom. "Why do I not postpone publication . . . until further experience has given me proof?" (Freud, 1925, p. 248). Freud calls on his collaborators, who now exist in greater numbers than before, to undertake the task of gathering evidence.

As Fliegel points out, this invitation was answered by his women students, Duetsch and Lampl-de Groot, who published clinical material supporting Freud's position, whereas Jones and Fenichel, two men students, differed with Freud. Fliegel tells us further that the Horney controversy simply vanished from the publications of the orthodox Freudian movement. Jones's disagreement with Freud was never recanted, but Freud simply dismissed the controversy in subsequent publications. Jones's biography of Freud contains only cryptic and bland references to the controversy. Fliegel contrasts this with Jones's detailed treatment of other controversies—for example, over how to proofread the *International Journal of Psychoanalysis!* Jones is also quite bland about the subsequent career of Horney, noting simply that in 1932 Horney was on her way to New York, and ignoring the fact that she was also on her way out of the Freudian school.

For her part, Horney, whose rich clinical observations had been given such short shrift by Freud, was much more polemical in her next publication on the subject, her famous 1926 paper on the flight from womanhood (Horney, 1926/1967). In this paper she clearly formulates the concept of womb envy on the part of boys, a concept that has led to considerable work on the part of anthropologists, beginning with Margaret Mead (1949). Horney also now personalizes the controversy. She pays tribute to Freud's genius, but finds it not surprising that as a man he has difficulty understanding women. This paper contains a table in which, in parallel columns, boys' fantasies about girls are compared with psychoanalysts' fantasies ("our views") about women. The resulting similarity is compelling evidence for the sexism that Horney was trying to describe in Freud's thinking.

FREUD AND MAINSTREAM PSYCHOLOGY OF SEX DIFFERENCES

In present-day mainstream academic psychology Freud's views on sex-role differences are generally criticized not only for their sexist bias but also for the assumption that sex roles are rooted in instinctual life. Freud's metapsychological constructs in which the sexual instinct creates identifications, incorporations, and introjections of parental figures out of the instinctive dread of castration (either threatened in the case of boys or already accomplished in the case of girls) are criticized for their vagueness of meaning. Two influential alternative lines of theorizing about the differences have been offered: a social learning theory (Mischel, 1966) and a cognitive-developmental approach (Kohlberg, 1966). As we shall see from an analysis of both of these approaches, difficulties arise in both that can be traced to the same hard place that Freud occupied: an inadequate theory of emotions as central to the life of a social human being.

Social Learning Theory

Mischel takes the position that behavior that is labeled "identification" by Freud and "imitation" by learning theorists is essentially the same phenomenon with two different names. Both imitation and identification

> refer to the tendency for a person to reproduce the actions, attitudes and emotional responses exhibited by real-life or symbolic models. It is of considerable theoretical importance that observational learning can take place without direct reinforcement to the observer. A wide range of direct and indirect imitative responses may be elicited, or inhibited, both in the presence and in the absence of a model. (1966, p. 57)

This position clearly assumes a preexisting social-emotional tie between the observer and the model, on which the "tendency" to imitate is founded. Not only the nature but the very existence of this tie is left unspecified. But it is precisely the bond between the "observer" and the "model" that Freud was trying to specify as resulting from the workings of the sexual instinct.

Empirical studies done under the theoretical guidance of social learning theory have produced results that Freud could equally well have predicted. Children learn under conditions of nurturance and also under conditions in which the model has the power to punish or reward. "Anaclitic" identifications, as well as "identification with the aggressor," are both powerful stimulants to learning.

Social learning theory has also produced studies that offer empirical confirmation for the notion that a model will be imitated if it is powerful, even if it is also of the opposite sex.

> It becomes clear why cultures—all of which vary in the degree to which one sex or the other controls valuable resources—produce differential degrees of cross-sex behavior. When females have markedly less access to powerful rewards than males, they may emulate male behavior to the degree to which such cross-sex behavior is tolerated. (Michel, 1966, p. 58)

This is surely a behaviorist's version of penis envy, emphasizing the social conditions that give rise to it, specifically the emotional ties that create the "tendency" for emulation. The "tendency to emulate," the "sexual instinct," and the "social-emotional nature" of human beings are all different phrasings for a mostly unknown "given" that psychologists are forced to assume.

Cognitive-Developmental Theory

Kohlberg's approach (1966) starts with cognition. Sex-role attitudes are essentially cognitive in that they are "rooted in the child's concept of *physical things*—the bodies of himself and others" (p. 82, italics added). Kohlberg explicitly models his approach after Piaget's description of the developmental progression in the child's "basic cognitive organization of the physical world" (p. 83). It should be noted that in order to accommodate to Piaget's system, Kohlberg treats the child's body only as a physical object, thereby ignoring the basic distinction between attitudes toward the physical world and attitudes toward social relationships. Kohlberg contrasts his theory with Mischel's as follows:

> The social-learning syllogism is: "I want rewards, I am rewarded for doing boy things, therefore I want to be a boy." In contrast, a cognitive theory assumes this sequence: "I am a boy, therefore I want to do boy things, therefore the opportunity to do boy things (and to gain approval for doing them) is rewarding." (p. 89)

Kohlberg does not ignore motivational and emotional factors in sex-role identity; he relies on motives of effectance and competence (White, 1959), and the "need to preserve a stable and positive self-image" (p. 88). As he puts the contrast between his theory and Freud's, gender identity is not "determined by instinctual wishes and gratifications, but [is] part of the general process of conceptual growth" (p. 98). Kohlberg further suggests that the child "engages in 'spontaneous' evaluations of his own worth to himself, and that he has 'natural' tendencies to seek worth and to compare his worth with that of others and to evaluate others" (p. 108). Once the cognitive judgment of gender identity is formed, then the child will value his or her gender because he or she values the self. The child identifies with the like-sex parent on this same basis.

Although Kohlberg has little use for psychoanalytic theory in general, he here seems to be making use of a concept much like that of primary narcissism, a very early and orthodox Freudian concept. The "natural" tendency to ascribe worth to the self that Kohlberg postulates is an innate process, similar to primary narcissism. As we have seen, Freud's concept of primary narcissism was partly the result of his failure to distinguish between the "ego" and the "self." The concept of an ego in love with itself was unsatisfactory to Hartmann (1951), who corrected it by introducing the additional notion of a conflict-free, autonomous ego. One version of this unconflicted ego is White's concept (1959) of the self enjoying its own powers. All of these concepts—"natural self-worth," a "conflict-free ego," and the "effectance motive"—carry theorizing away from the concept of an infant as a social being, born into a social interaction with its caretaker, and evolving a self that is ineluctably social even in its most individuated or narcissistic forms (Lewis, 1980).

Feminist psychologists who are also in mainstream academia understandably tend to discard Freud as either too fanciful or too biological. In their monumental *Psychology of Sex Differences,* Maccoby and Jacklin (1974), for example, ignore Freud. They cite him only once, then only to notice that he "stumbled" in his view that there are "anaclitic" and "defensive" identifications. But Maccoby and Jacklin may be laboring under the same androcentric bias that governed Freud. They accept the genetic basis for aggression in males (via the established fact that there is genetic control of differing sex hormones). This line of reasoning would also directly suggest a genetic basis for maternal behavior (via the same route of hormonal control). Although Maccoby and Jacklin have "no doubt that women throughout the world are perceived to be the nurturant sex" (p. 215), they do not accord the notion that nurturant behavior in women is genetically based the status of an equal hypothesis with the genetic control of aggression in males. Maccoby and Jacklin also conclude that the greater sociability of women as compared with men is a "myth." This conclusion is, in my opinion, premature, as I have documented within their own survey (Lewis, 1976). In any case, Maccoby and Jacklin's survey of sex differences makes little reference to the role of social and political forces governing the psychological development of the two sexes, except to indicate their belief that it is no "historical accident" that "males have occupied the high-status positions in the large majority of human social groupings" (p. 368). In this view, they share Freud's biologism.

Freud's work on sex differences has thus clearly influenced modern academia, if only as a foil against which to formulate empirical approaches. It is not clear why condescending disclaimers of the value of Freudian interpretations have become so obligatory among experimenters, especially since the theoretical problems he confronted are still with us today.

FREUDIAN INTERPRETATIONS: INSIGHTS INTO GENDER IDENTITY

Freud's most enduring contribution to our understanding of sex differences comes from his insight into the extent to which primary-process transformations of conflicted feelings govern human attitudes about sex and sex differences. With this powerful instrument for un-

raveling conflicted feelings, psychoanalysis can predict with some success certain universals of experience for the two sexes. As Jahoda (1977)
puts it, "every child has to discover anew the existence and meaning of
morphological sex differences" (p. 88) within the context of passionate
attachments to its nuclear family. The success of anthropologists in
using Freudian concepts to predict the relationship between cultural
forces and attitudes toward sex will be more fully detailed in Chapter 9.
At this point it will be useful to outline some of the ways in which
attitudes of men and women are determined by their gender identity.

The linguistic and social connotations of the term "gender identity"
suggest that sexual identity is a primary-process transformation of affects and self-images formed by each of us in interaction with our earliest caretakers. "Gender," as distinct from sex, also suggests that identification of oneself as male or female is itself a complicated part of the
socialization process and not an automatic consequence of chromosomal
endowment. This supposition in turn suggests that adult heterosexual
gender preference (like homosexuality) is the outcome of a long developmental process in which primary-process transformation, for instance, anaclitic and defensive identifications, play a decisive part.

Although all these concepts are implicit and explicit in his writings
on sex differences, Freud never actually used the term "gender identity." This term was first used by Stoller (1968) in his book about people
with chromosomal sex abnormalities. Psychoanalysts and psychologists
have welcomed the term, since it helps to keep some of the manifold
meanings of sex role disentangled.

In the sense that growing up in sexually different bodies inevitably
produces psychological differences in the acculturation process, anatomy is one determinant of destiny. Although the term "acculturation
process" has a modern ring, and although Freud actually talked more
about unreconstructed instincts being constantly opposed by culture,
Freud's basic assumption was that differences in the acculturation process were based on the sex difference. In his system primary-process
transformations were bound to be different for the self of the two sexes
because of intrinsic differences in the parent–child relationship. The
many experimental studies now demonstrating a sex difference in the
mother–infant interaction are clearly a confirmation of this basic Freudian assumption. Sex differences in the mother–infant interaction must
influence the course of subsequent acculturation in some universal
ways.

One of these predictable universals comes from the fact that women
have a same-sex first caretaker, whereas men have an opposite-sex first
caretaker as the first "object" of passionate attachment. Margaret Mead

(1949) picked up the implications of this universal, suggesting that the boy's "earliest experience of self is one in which he is forced, in the relationship to his mother, to realize himself as different, as a creature unlike his mother" (p. 167). Lynn (1961) developed this point in a behavioral mode, suggesting that girls have only to learn a "lesson" in mother-person emulation, whereas boys have to learn to differentiate the gender of the self from that of the first caretaker and then to "solve the problem" of father-person identification. Lynn suggested that the consequences for developmental events are different from Freud's predictions. For girls, the substructure of identity comes from assimilating "same-sex" in imitation of a personal relationship; for boys, identity involves more complicated cognitive events: restructuring of the perceptual field and abstracting principles of identification.

There is still another universal of experience stemming from the fact that the first caretaker is opposite-sex for boys and same-sex for girls. Boys' very early frustrations at the hands of their mothers form a substratum of experience when the time comes in adulthood for them to find a person of the opposite sex. Horney (1932/1967) suggests that the little boy judges his genital to be too small for his mother's vagina: "His original dread of women is not castration anxiety at all, but . . . the menace to his self-respect" (p. 142). Horney is careful to make the point that dread is not an inevitable characteristic of a boy's relationship to the opposite sex, only a frequent stress point, on which later noxious events can build. In contrast, little girls' interest in their fathers occurs at a time when they are much older. Their relationship to their fathers usually does not bear the imprint of earliest nurturance; on the contrary, experiences with father occur when the girl's self is quite well formed, and disappointments with father can be better borne by a self already well developed. Similarly, later disappointments in heterosexual relationships carry fewer scars of very ancient battles fought with mother.

Taken together with the more recent evidence of profound sex differences in the earliest mother–infant interaction, with boys being more difficult to pacify (Moss, 1974), the universal circumstance of same-sex versus cross-sex nurturant figures suggests that boys should have greater identity problems. Findings from our own culture support this prediction (Lewis, 1976). The point has not (to my knowldege) been studied in other cultures, but there are many instances of cultural encouragement for men to be homosexual reported in the literature (e.g., the berdache).

One of the most significant and puzzling findings of experimental studies of the mother–infant interaction that have developed from the questions raised about anatomy and destiny is the sex difference in vulnerability to maternal deprivation (Sackett, 1974). Males have been shown to be much more vulnerable to maternal deprivation not only in adult sexual capacity but also in a variety of other social behaviors. Although the evidence from our own acculturated species is less unequivocal than that from nonhuman mammals, there is more than a suggestion that human male infants are more subject to "inconsolable states" (Moss, 1974), and that maternal deprivation has a more clearly harmful effect on men than on women (Bayley & Schaefer, 1964). These experimental findings speak to the possibility of some intrinsic, genetic-hormonal differences between the sexes that may render females more resistant to the psychological stress of maternal deprivation.

Another line of investigation into the mother–infant interaction suggests that nonhuman mammal mothers not only can differentiate the sex of their pups but treat their male pups more "harshly." On the human level, there are studies that suggest that mothers have a harder time establishing a smooth interaction with their boy infants (Moss, 1974). The latter finding may itself be based, of course, on differences in mothers' attitudes toward the two genders, especially in a social system in which women are devalued. Differences in the symbolic meaning of boy and girl neonates to their parents have been demonstrated experimentally (e.g., Rubin, Provenzano, & Luria, 1974). Girl and boy infants are differently perceived in the eyes of their beholders (girls being perceived as "softer"). This does not preclude the possibility that girl infants actually do bring something genetically different into the infant–caretaker interaction. Their smoother interaction with their same-sex caretakers may make for a closer bond between the self and mother. In turn, this closer bond may interact with women's social inferiority to foster women's proneness to states of shame (Lewis, 1976).

Another predictable universal of gender differences in sexual attitudes is the greater difficulty intrinsic for men in adult heterosexual intercourse. Wide-ranging explanations, using primary-process transformations of the emotional conflicts evoked by this circumstance, have included differences in men's and women's anxieties during intercourse (Horney, 1932/1967) and characterological sex differences based on these differing anxieties (Fromm, 1943). Differential modes of experiencing the world, such as Erikson's (1964) "inner" and "outer" space, have also been suggested. A brief review of some of these uses of Freudian interpretation suggests the richness of his insight into human sexual behavior.

That intercourse is intrinsically more difficult for men than for women is illuminated by the contrast between ourselves and nonhuman primates, for whom the estrus cycle still controls both male as well as female sexual arousal. The loss of estrus in the human species has brought intercourse much more under social than hormonal control. It has also resulted in the loss of a failsafe stimulus. Yet intercourse for men is still the same three-step process that can be seen among mammals: arousal-erection; intromission; ejaculation-orgasm (Beach, 1965). A man's failure to have an erection or to maintain it prevents intercourse; no such burden of responsibility for intercourse is carried by women. A woman has only to be present and willing to permit penetration. A man must be aroused, a state not necessarily under his conscious control. The act of intercourse is thus more difficult for men and easier for women. Her orgasm, moreover, plays no role in her fertilization, whereas a man's ejaculation-orgasm is necessary for fertilization.

As Horney (1932/1967) put it:

> The man is actually obliged to go on proving his manhood to the woman. There is no analogous necessity for her. Even if she is frigid she can engage in sexual intercourse and conceive and bear a child. She performs her part merely by *being*, without any *doing*—a fact that has always filled men with admiration and resentment. The man, on the other hand, has to *do* something in order to fulfill himself. The ideal of "efficiency" is a typical masculine ideal. (p. 145)

The gestalt of feelings and attitudes governing experience in sexual intercourse is thus "phallocentric" for men. The intruder in a man's sexual experience is the fear of his failure to have and maintain an erection. Fromm (1943) describes how the fear of impotence in a male increases his need for "mastery," an attitude that coupled with resentment against women can readily turn into domination and rape. In contrast, women's attitudes toward sex are more embedded in the framework of possible maternity. Women's sexual experience has as a frequent intruder the image of herself as mother, with both the pleasurable and the fearful consequences of pregnancy.

Cross-cultural evidence suggests the accuracy of some of these interpretations of universal experience. Ford and Beach (1951) showed that "love charms are much more often employed by men than by women" (pp. 108–109). Their survey of sexual behavior also showed that the majority of cultures studied believed that men should take the initiative in intercourse. This belief must in part reflect the acknowledgment of a necessity. Margaret Mead (1949) makes the point that

> the male who has learned various mechanical ways to stimulate his sexual specificity in order to copulate with a woman he does not at the moment desire is doing far more violence to his nature than a female who needs only receive a male. (p. 210)

Horney's distinction between *being* and *doing* has stimulated a great deal of anthropological research on the development of sex roles (see, e.g., Chodorow, 1971). The distinction between being and doing has an analogue in the fact that women's gender identity is at lesser risk of malformation than men's, and it may be one component of the sex difference in proneness to depression and paranoia that was traced in Volume 1.

Another important primary-process resultant of the caretaker's gender is the way in which men's aggressions against women are fostered and rationalized by their relationship to their mothers. Dinnerstein (1977) has shown that the subordinate position of women is fostered by a family structure in which both boys and girls are predominantly reared by their mother: Boys' aggressions are especially exaggerated by the circumstance of earliest rearing by an opposite-sex caretaker. Baumrind (1980), summarizing new directions in socialization research, emphasizes the importance and usefulness of studies of one-sided rearing versus "parenting." Chodorow (1978) has also made use of Freudian concepts in her cross-cultural studies of the *reproduction* of mothering.

Erikson (1964) raised the question of human survival in his paper on womanhood and inner space. Erikson begins this essay by pointing with alarm to the fact that men have brought the species to the brink of destruction, and suggests that women may have to save it.

> Maybe if women could gain the determination to represent publicly what they have always stood for privately in evolution and history (realism of upbringing, resourcefulness in peace-keeping and devotion to healing), they might well add an ethically restraining, because truly supranational, power to politics in the widest sense. (p. 604)

Finally, as I suggested in Chapter 4, the recent work on psychological androgyny may reasonably be regarded as an outgrowth of Freudian interpretations. Freud carefully distinguished (as nearly always, with clinical accuracy) between masculine and feminine personality and the gender of a person's sexual object-choice. Men homosexuals, he observed, are by no means always feminine in personality, nor are women homosexuals always masculine. Present-day work on psychological androgyny (e.g., Bem, 1976), correcting earlier unipolar concepts of masculinity–femininity, represents an extension of Freud's view that masculinity and femininity are complicated resultants of emotional interactions with significant adults and significant cultural values.

The growing literature on psychological androgyny now questions whether masculinity and femininity are two poles of a single personality dimension. It suggests, rather, that masculinity and femininity may be independent personality dimensions, or else orthogonally related. Even more important, androgynous sex-role identity is now considered to be more adaptive than conventional sex-role typing, since it allows greater flexibility of behavior. Thus, for example, androgynous women were found to be more nonconforming than feminine women; correspondingly, androgynous men were found to be more nurturant than masculine men (Bem, 1975; Bem, Martyna, & Watson, 1976). Another study showed that in an experimental situation designed to elicit expressive behavior, androgynous men gazed at the person to whom they were speaking and smiled more often (when not speaking) than did masculine-typed men (LaFrance & Carmen, 1980). Thus, androgynous people are adding to their repertory of useful behaviors rather than showing inconsistent and perhaps pathological "cross-sex" behavior.

PSYCHOANALYSIS AND FEMINISM: A RAPPROCHEMENT

As has been apparent throughout this chapter, feminist issues have always been intrinsic in Freud's work, although clouded by his androcentrism and misogyny. A critique of the existing patterns of marriage was explicit in Freud's first descriptions of the suffering of hysterical women. Here is an example of Freud's (1908b) sympathetic clinical description of women's plight:

> Let us, for instance, consider the very common case of a woman who does not love her husband because, owing to the conditions under which she entered marriage, she has no reason to love him, but who wants very much to love him, because that alone corresponds to the ideal of marriage to which she has been brought up. She will in that case suppress every impulse which would express the truth and contradict her endeavors to fulfill her ideal, and she will make special efforts to play the part of a loving, affectionate and attentive wife. The outcome of this self-suppression will be a neurotic illness; and this neurosis will in a short time have taken revenge on the unloved husband and have caused him as much lack of satisfaction and worry as would have resulted from an acknowledgement of the true state of affairs. This example is completely typical of what a neurosis achieves. (p. 203)

Feminist issues in Freud's work were entangled not only with his androcentrism, but with the deeper question of the relationship between society and the individual. Having first observed the noxious effects of sexual repression, Freud then justified repression by considering the individual's sexual repression to be the necessary basis for the existence of civilization. The principal psychoanalytic revisionists, Adler, Horney, Fromm, and Reich, used socialist principles as a basis of their critique of civilization. Distinguishing the effects of more and less benign social orders, they explicitly disagreed with Freud that all societies are based on the suppression of sexuality. They understood the interaction between sex-roles and family dynamics as occurring within the framework of an exploitative and competitive society. The actual difference in power between men and women was seen as an important factor underlying primary-process fantasies about the "natural" sex roles of men and women.

Both Fromm and Reich, for example, characterize the patriarchal family as a reflection in miniature of exploitative power in a societal background, and suggest that, in this sense, the family is a transmission belt for attitudes that derogate women. Reich is most explicit in restricting Freud's critique of civilization to civilization's present forms. He follows Engels in assuming that the oppression of women makes its appearance at the same time as the establishment of an oppressing class.

Most important of all, however, both Fromm and Reich share the conviction, which Freud did not have, that the abolition of exploitation would free human beings from the character deformations they now suffer as its consequence. Fromm (1955), for example, envisages the "sane society" as one in which the central value is human growth, not the use of human beings as commodities. In such a society, individuals would develop so that conflicts between the self and others are minimal. The implication of this view is that human beings of both sexes have a "natural tendency" toward peaceable relationships with each other. This is in effect a theory that postulates the social nature of human beings, with attachment emotions basic to their existence. We shall return to this question in Chapter 8.

Psychoanalytically sophisticated political criticism of the social order has found recent expression in important works by feminists on rape (Brownmiller, 1975) and on incest (Herman, 1981). Brownmiller's study makes clear that rape has been an instrument by which warring societies reward their soldiers and at the same time perpetuate the oppression of women. Herman points out that father–daughter incest is by far the most frequent form of sexual exploitation. She interprets this fact as a reflection of patriarchal power, and as a means of perpetuating it. Both these studies make use of Freudian interpretation, while explicitly disavowing the content of Freud's views on women.

In recent times, several attempts have been made to effect an explicit rapprochement between psychoanalysis and feminism. My own attempt (Lewis, 1976) was made from the psychoanalyst's side and it built on the revisions suggested by the Freudian "left." Mitchell (1974), speaking from the political-feminist side, has made generous use of a Freudian revisionist, Lacan (1975). Mitchell draws on Lacan's criticisms of Freudian metapsychology to help bring feminism and psychoanalysis together.

Lacan is particularly critical of Freud's metapsychology for its nonaffective formulations. In Lacan's system, the data of psychoanalysis derive from the dialogue between two selves (thus, in my view, reflecting the state of their emotional relatedness). Psychoanalysis is therefore a "science of mirages" that has developed a special language for these emotional transactions. As pointed out in Volume 1, this is a felicitous phrasing of Freud's concept of primary-process transformations of emotional conflict. Lacan brings his concept of the dialogue into line with more recent linguistic theories of universal grammar, criticizing Freud's concept of the inchoate unconscious because it could better be understood as structured like a language. Mitchell suggests that the psychoanalytic concept of the unconscious is the concept of mankind's transmission and inheritance of social and cultural laws. In each unconscious are all mankind's "ideas" of history. Understanding the laws of the unconscious thus amounts to a start in understanding how ideology functions. Of particular significance, of course, is the ideology of women's inferiority.

Although Mitchell effected this bridge by a considerable looseness in her handling of Freud's writings (Fliegel, 1982), the effort she has made to reinterpret Freud has met with some acceptance among feminist psychologists and psychoanalysts. Most important, her work pinpoints the place where Freud's work needs revision: a thoroughgoing replacement of Freud's metapsychology by a theory based on human social and emotional relatedness.

CHAPTER 6

Mistakes and Jokes
"Primary Process": The Problem of the Relation between Cognition and Affect

Freud extended his use of the concept of "primary process" in two books after *The Interpretation of Dreams* (1900), a book on everyday mistakes (1901b) and a book on jokes (1905a). These two books turn our attention away from the problem of the social nature of human nature back to the narrower problem of the relation between cognition and affect. As we shall see in this chapter, these two issues are related. They become connected in the problem of how to understand the obviously high level of intellectual functioning that can produce the "compromise" content of mistakes, and the even more dazzling intellectual feats that are the "joke work." These intellectual feats occur under the press of maintaining affectional ties.

A view of human nature that regards it as individualistic concentrates on the consequences of frustrated individual needs. This is the version of Freud's theory that he formally espoused. Fear and anger are the "negative" emotions from which human cognition starts. In such a view, the negative emotions are all-powerful; the role of reason is to tame them or help us outgrow them. Cognitions developed under the press of negative affect are "regressive," even hallucinatory, as, for example, the dreams that occur in sleep. "Primary process," in this view, is primitive, and to be replaced by secondary or rational processes.

In contrast, a view of human nature that starts with attachment sees the positive emotions as appropriate to attachment and the negative emotions as appropriate to threatened or broken attachment; both, however, push for its maintenance. Positive emotions are not only appropriate to attachment but also facilitative of cognitions in general. Positive emotions, coalesced in a positively toned, competent self, facilitate the development of cognitions in general. The role of cognition is not just to curb emotions since these are not necessarily interferences with cognition that need to be outgrown. Thoughts, moreover, do not merely bind or reduce feelings, but they can also express and enhance feeling, especially in congruent ideas and images, that is, in symbolic or metaphoric form. Positive emotions, coalesced in a positively toned "self," facilitate the development of complicated, sophisticated ways of expressing conflicted feelings, as well as complicated thoughts. This is a version of Freudian theory compatible with his clinical observations, especially those in the books on mistakes and jokes.

As we saw in Chapters 1 and 2, and previously in Volume 1, Freud described clinically how primary-process transformations occur during "undischarged" states of shame and guilt, and then chose "instincts" as the core of his theory. I have more recently suggested that shame and guilt are affective-cognitive states that arise in broken attachment and press toward its restoration (Lewis, 1981). The thoughts thus arising express both sides of feeling—the forbidding and the forbidden—in a primary-process transformation that effects a "compromise" and keeps the self attached. For such a complicated social maneuver it is not surprising that the thoughts evoked can be of a high level of cognitive complexity. This is particularly apparent not only in some dreams and in everyday mistakes, but in jokes that make use of exquisite subtleties of thought.

Freud's descriptions of the categories of primary-process transformations include condensation, displacement, and symbolism as well as hallucinatory images. The first three categories clearly involve complex intellectual functioning. Freud was aware of the problem posed by the cognitive complexity of primary process, although he never directly addressed it. For example, as we saw in Chapter 1, he quoted with approbation Scherner's view that dreams, freed from the restraints of reason, are "productive" creations rather than merely regressive. In his summary of the varieties of primary process, "regression to images," which refers to the hallucinatory wish in dreams, is specifically said *not* to be the main point of dream work. What has remained since Freud's day is his descriptive account of primary process that sometimes involves dazzling intellectual feats, and a theoretical account, more often quoted, in which primary process is synonymous with the unknowable id.

Although he called some jokes "brilliant," Freud could not incorporate this observation at all into his theoretical system. Because jokes are social, he understood them to require "intelligibility" (1905a, p. 179) for their effect, but he did not inquire further how they come to be brilliant. On the contrary, he relegated jokes to the realm of inessential play, whereas dreams (which are unintelligible) express more profound needs. One important issue that lies buried in this downgrading of the function of jokes is the assumption that play is relatively unimportant *because* it is not conflictual.

As Freud described the process, the high level of intellectual functioning in some jokes depends upon the power of both positive and negative affects, which have been evoked simultaneously, to produce congruent, double-sided thoughts. (These double-sided thoughts can also enhance the affects.) As Freud puts it, jokes depend upon the "ambiguity of words and the multiplicity of conceptual relations" (1905a, p. 172). The ambiguities and complexities of conceptual relations reflect ambivalence. They transform it, however, by creating new analogies that now (appropriately) express an incongruity. Incongruity evokes laughter, one of the universal affective expressions of attachment. A joke's brilliance thus inheres in its use of appropriate cognitive symbols to reflect ambivalence in an incongruity that dissolves ambivalence in laughter.

The fate of Freud's *Psychopathology of Everyday Life* (1901b) has been very different from that of his *Jokes and Their Relation to the Unconscious* (1905). The former work is one of Freud's most widely read; moreover, it was constantly revised and expanded with fresh examples by Freud himself. The book on *Jokes* is perhaps Freud's least read (Jones, 1954). Generally it is treated by the public and by professionals as a tangential work. Freud himself speaks of it as a work that led him temporarily from his main path (1915–1916). This is perhaps because the distinguishing phenomena of jokes—their sophisticated linguistic techniques, their positive affect, and their social character—are particularly difficult to fit into Freud's metapsychology. In any case, these two books are the major works in which Freud confronted the relation between affect and cognition in normal, everyday waking life as distinct from dreams and neurotic symptoms.

THE PSYCHOPATHOLOGY OF EVERYDAY LIFE

Freud explicitly placed a "high theoretical value" (1910, p. 38) on his discovery that affects can distort cognition in normal, everyday waking life as well as in dreams and neurotic symptoms. His book on mistakes demonstrated to him that "repression and the formation of sub-stitutes can occur even under healthy conditions" (1910, p. 38). The extent to which Freud's observations about motivated everyday mis-takes have become folk wisdom is reflected in a new English word, "parapraxis," which Freud's translators coined to categorize emo-tionally motivated cognitive distortions.

Freud's observational account of his own parapraxes was based, like the book on dreams, on his own experience and introspection. In his account he is very cautious about the extent to which motivational con-flict can account for any specific distortion. He explicitly did not chal-lenge the academic psychologists' laws on memory and perception. "Perhaps it is superfluous to remark," he wrote, "that the conditions which psychologists assume to be necessary for reproducing and for forgetting and which they look for in certain relations and dispositions, are not inconsistent [with Freud's explanations]" (1901b, p.7).

Freud's view of the parapraxes, moreover, was *not* that there was no basis for them in "circulatory disturbances" or "general functional disturbances of the cerebrum" (1901b, p.21), but that the motivational factor that he called repression was an important and neglected addition to the total circumstances. By the time of his *Five Lectures* (1910), he was espousing a strict determinism in psychological laws that made it seem that *all* parapraxes were the result of repression. This was, however, more an expression of his view that "instinct" or motivations govern all behavior than it was an overgeneralization about parapraxes.

Let us look closely at the first example of parapraxis in the *The Psychopathology of Everyday Life* (1901b), Freud's "motivated" forgetting of the proper name, Signorelli. This is one of Freud's most famous clinical examples, partly because he used it often. Signorelli was the artist who painted the Orvieto cathedral frescoes, *Four Last Things: Death, Judgment, Heaven and Hell.* In addition to suddenly forgetting the name, Signorelli, which he knew well, Freud found himself thinking of two substitute names, knowing they were incorrect. His explanation includes the associative process by which these two names occurred to him as itself driven by the same underlying motivation as the sudden, unexpected forgetting.

As we read the text it becomes clear that the affective states of shame and guilt with which Freud was struggling are not explicitly named by him although the reader has no trouble identifying them as the background "disturbances." As we saw in the analysis of the Irma dream (Chapter 1), Freud needed his own stream of associative connec-tions to lead him to these background affective states. He himself was unaware of them at the time of the forgetting of Signorelli's name.

Although, as we shall see in a moment, he concludes that he must have been under the influence of his feelings over a patient's suicide, he tells us only that his thoughts were driven to turn away from this "melancholy event" and as a result he forgot Signorelli, and misremembered Botticelli and Boltraffio. The clinical account is thus rich in tracing the associative connections leading to the forgetting and the substitution without explicitly tracing each connection back to affective states of shame and guilt. This, again, the reader can do more easily than Freud could.

Freud tells us that when he was driving in the company of a stranger from Ragusa to a place in Herzegovina, the subject of Italian painters came up and Freud asked his companion if he had ever been to Orvieto and seen the famous frescoes by . . . The substitute names Botticelli and Boltraffio came to his mind, not because Botticelli was any more familiar to him than Signorelli—Boltraffio is a fact less familiar to him—but because of some intrinsic connection between these names and the same affective disturbance that caused him to forget.

As Freud analyzed his own associative connections (again, as in the Irma dream, post hoc), they led him to his patient's suicide. He remembered that right before the subject of Italian painters came up, he had been telling the stranger about the attitudes of Turkish patients in *Bos*nia and *Her*zegovina toward their doctors. "There is great confidence in doctors such that if one has to say the patient will die, the reply is: 'Herr (signor) . . . if he could be saved, I know you would save him.'" Freud also remembered wanting to tell the stranger another anecdote he was also thinking of about Turks in Bosnia and Herzegovina:

> They place a higher value on sexual enjoyment than on anything else, and in the event of sexual disorders they are plunged in a despair which contrasts strangely with their resignation towards the threat of death. (1901b, p. 3)

Freud had suppressed telling this anecdote because of the "delicacy of the topic." He also turned away from

> pursuing the thoughts which might have arisen in my mind from the topic of "death and sexuality." On this occasion I was still under the influence of a piece of news that had reached me a few weeks before while I was making a brief stay at *Traf*oi [a hamlet in the Tyrol]. *A patient over whom I had taken a great deal of trouble had put an end to his life on account of an incurable sexual disorder. I know for certain that this melancholy event and everything related to it was not recalled to my conscious memory during my journey to Herzegovina. But the similarity between Trafoi and Bol*traf*fio forces me to assume that this reminiscence in spite of my attention being deliberately diverted from it was brought into operation at the time* [of the conversation]. (1901b, pp. 3–4, italics added)

Freud's description of the process by which the forgetting occurred emphasizes the element of volition. He wanted to forget something—

which he labels only as the theme of death and sexuality. *"I forgot the one thing against my will,* while I wanted to forget *the other thing intentionally"* (p. 4, Freud's italics). "By a sort of compromise they [the substitute names] remind me just as much of what I wanted to forget as what I wanted to remember." In this account, with its emphasis on volition, Freud sounds as if the forgetting and substitution were not only a compromise but a punishment for what he wanted to forget. But his reference to guilt and shame is implicit rather than overt.

The account of how each detail of the cognitive content is linked to details of both the forgetting and the substitution is very full; Freud clarifies it in a well-known diagram (Figure 1) in which he spells out the "picture puzzle" or "rebus."

The laws of cognitive connection employed by this rebus are the familiar associations in laws of similarity and contiguity still current. The rebus, moreover, is an example of a complicated primary-process transformation. In addition to the laws of association that are at work, there is in operation an emotional congruity between Freud's state of mind and the theme of the Signorelli painting. The congruity between the subject of the Orvieto frescoes—death and judgment—and Freud's state of mind over his patient's suicide is not mentioned until a footnote in the next chapter, where Freud tells us that "repressed thoughts on the

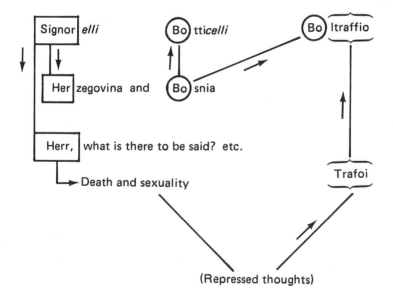

FIGURE 1. Freud's Rebus.

subject of death and sexual life [are] by no means remote from the topic of the frescoes at Orvieto" (p. 13).

Freud's use of the theme "death and sexuality" to describe his repressed thoughts is much less affectively loaded than it might have been had he referred specifically to his shame and guilt over his patient's suicide. By implication, however, the Turks who have implicit conficence in their doctors are a bit foolish. This is a ridiculing stance that Freud allowed himself when he first spoke to his traveling companion. The next train of thought (which he did not speak) reminded him of "death and sexuality" among the (foolish) Turks. This could have resonated, although he did not remember it until later, with his thoughts of the (foolish) patient who killed himself over sex. As he then turned his thoughts to painting in Italy, the (Signorelli) painting came to mind (a much admired masterpiece) and Freud suddenly experienced the discomfiture of not being able to remember! Once again, a specific connection between this uncomfortable forgetting and Freud's feeling of responsibility (guilt) for the death of his patient and/or his feeling of shame at failure to prevent it is not explicit.

Each of the chapters in *The Psychopathology of Everyday Life* takes up a specific kind of parapraxis, reflecting Freud's careful clinical description of the circumstances besides "motivation" that are involved in each. A great number and variety of parapraxes are described in chapters on loss of well-memorized material, childhood memories and falsification, slips of the tongue, slips of the pen, misprints, forgetting of impressions and of intentions, losing things, breaking things, and accident proness. As we have seen, some of the most moving examples come from Freud's own shame and guilt over possible misdiagnosis. Freud's theoretical formulations are, as usual, not phrased directly in terms of unbearable states of shame and guilt but in terms of "incompletely suppressed psychical material, which although pushed away by consciousness, has nevertheless not been robbed of all capacity for expressing itself" (1910, p. 279).

The impact of Freud's *Psychopathology of Everyday Life* has been enormous, beginning with its bringing the Rat Man to Freud as a patient. Among the general public, "motivated" mistakes, slips, forgettings, accidents are now an accepted, often amusing, fact of life. Among academic psychologists, the attempt to replicate Freud's observations and to bring them under systematic inquiry has resulted in literally thousands of experimental studies, with mixed and sometimes disappointing results. During the 1940s and 1950s the "New Look's" studies of perception, learning, and forgetting at first seemed to promise "verification" of Freud's emphasis on the power of emotions in ordinary, everyday human thinking. Soon an era of disappointment set in, when the ordinary laws of cognition seemed to be quietly accounting for some too hastily interpreted "Freudian" results. Many of these results were reinterpreted as "artifacts" of insufficient attention to cognitive laws (see, e.g., Eriksen, 1963). Proponents of such "cognitive" determinants as the familiarity of words (versus their "taboo" quality), the effects of "expectancy set," or of "response bias" seemed for a while to be winning important points over the proponents of "repression."

More recently, the critics of the New Look have been subjected to some criticism themselves: namely, that concepts of "set" and "bias" also imply unconscious determinants (Erdelyi, 1974). Erdelyi suggests that an information-processing model may account for the "selectivity" of perceptual vigilance and defense. Recently, Bowlby (1980) has attempted a merger of information-processing and psychoanalytic theories of repression and defense, a point to which we shall shortly return.

It should be remembered that in his descriptive accounts of parapraxes Freud never discounted the "ordinary" laws of cognition. What he described were the special instances in which they were insufficient to account for a parapraxis. Experimental studies that pit cognitive and affective conditions against each other are not a test of Freud's descriptions of parapraxes.

It is impossible to do justice to the thousands of studies that have been done attempting to bring a "new (Freudian) look" to the fields of perception, learning, and thinking. The two massive surveys of the experimental literature on Freudian theory (Kline, 1971; Fisher & Greenberg, 1977) tend, on the whole, to find considerable support for Freud's clinical descriptions. Many studies often ingeniously confirm Freud's clinical observations about the importance of emotional determinants in normal human behavior. What remains to be understood is the process by which affect and cognition influence each other. Freud's theoretical stance in attacking this question was so biased in the direction of positing only the interfering effects of negative affects that the theoretical problems have not yet been adequately stated.

The work of Rapaport (1968) in attempting to systematize Freudian theory has tended to emphasize the aspect of Freudian theorizing that sharply differentiated between primary and secondary process as primitive and advanced, respectively. This leaves cognition and affect in their familiar adversary position, and makes it more difficult to apprehend how they work congruently.

A less well-known work along theoretical lines is Madison's (1961) careful study of Freud's theoretical and clinical writings in an effort to disentangle Freud's uses of the terms "repression" and "defense."

Freud himself ultimately assigned to "repression" the narrower meaning of amnesic loss, and resolved to use, instead, the broader term
"defense" of the ego; but he never actually gave up using the term
"repression" more broadly. Madison suggests that this is not the result
of a semantic inconsistency but of the deeper fact that both repression
and defense refer to an "interplay of force and counter-force" (p. 9).
Madison is thus calling attention to the interplay of emotions that is focal
in understanding behavior. Freud could not contain his observations in
a concept of cognitive loss but rather needed some theoretical concept of
an ego or, more accurately, of a self in an emotional dilemma. This is a
position similar to my own, which draws attention to the usefulness of a
focus on both the phenomenology and theory of states of shame and
guilt.

JOKES AND THEIR RELATION TO THE UNCONSCIOUS

In Freud's book on jokes, the narrowness of his conceptualizations
can be seen in even greater relief than in his work on parapraxes, since
by his own account jokes are a social process. Freud's book on jokes was
based partly on a collection of his favorite Jewish jokes that he himself
had compiled. His favorites were the jokes that had occasioned the
heartiest laughter. These jokes were of special interest to him because he
was familiar with the humiliations of being Jewish, and most admiring
of his compatriots' capacity to respond to such feelings with laughter.
Freud's other "subjective reason for taking up the problem of jokes"
(1900, p. 173) was also connected with a feeling of humiliation. He tells
us that uninformed people, on first hearing about the abundant use in
dreams of displacements and allusions, receive "an uncomfortable impression" (p. 173) and are inclined to think of his interpretations as a
joke. (It was Fliess in particular to whom Freud was responding.)
Freud's difficulty in not being taken seriously as an interpreter is a
reminder of similar attitudes that arise in evaluating the work of Lévi-
Strauss. Lévi-Strauss's insights into the elaborate cognitive processes by
which nonliterate people arrive at their myths and customs (see, e.g.,
the myth of the Wawilak sisters, Lewis, 1976) sometimes evoke wonder
as to whether the brilliance inheres in the people's reasoning or in Lévi-
Strauss! The joke in this instance expresses in laughter the chagrin of
recognizing that "primitive" people are at least as intellectually developed as, if not superior to, "civilized" peoples in some of their understanding of the world. Laughter, even in chagrin, is a pleasurable feeling—or at least it is less painful than humiliation. This was the major

point of Freud's interpretation of jokes: They "transform" humiliation and reproach into shared laughter—and they do so by very clever cognitive "techniques."

Freud's first illustration of how his own approach differs from that of his contemporaries is his treatment of what he terms a "brilliant" joke by Heine. One of Heine's characters, a poor lottery agent named Hirsch-Hyacinth boasts that the great Baron Rothschild treats him as an equal quite "famillionairely." As Freud points out, Hirsch-Hyacinth is a self-parody of Heine himself, whose rich uncle Salomon always treated him "a little famillionairely, as a poor relation" (1905a, p. 141). Freud's translation of this joke differs from that of Lipps and Heymans in that Freud supplements their essentially cognitive description with his own affective translation of the joke's "thoughts." Freud accepts both Lipp's and Heymans's notion that "bewilderment and illumination" are implicit in the hybrid joke-word. But he adds a translation of the implied affective content of Hirsch-Hyacinth's thoughts:

> "Rothschild treated me quite as his equal, quite familiarly—that is, so far as a millionaire can." "A rich man's condescension," we should add, "always involves something not quite pleasant for whoever experiences it."

Freud is thus describing the "unmistakable bitterness, which is understandable in a poor man faced by such great wealth" (p. 17). These feelings and thoughts, however, are not, so far, a joke. In the joke-word, what has "disappeared" is the "whole limitation added by the second sentence" (p. 18), that is, the feeling of humiliation. The joke-word, "famillionaire," moreover, is a composite of the two thoughts contained in the first sentence of Hirsch-Hyacinth's thought, as translated by Freud: " 'R. treated me quite familiarly, that is, so far as a millionaire can.' " In this composite the element, "so far as a millionaire *can*" has been lost (italics added), and the element "millionaire" has been retained. Although Freud does not explicitly say so, the composite word directs attention away from the (correct?) recognition of the impossibility that millionaires can really be equal (familiar) with poor relations. In this recognition, the gulf between the millionaire and his poor relation is an (objective?) circumstance that might even evoke some pity or scorn for millionaires. The joke replaces the bitterness of humiliation and scorn with laughter at both parties.

THE COGNITIVE COMPLEXITY OF JOKES

Freud distinguishes between jokes that have a "logical facade" and jokes that have a "nonsensical" appearance. In each category he analyzes the linguistic techniques that are involved. The central question he pursues in Socratic style is: How can a set of linguistic techniques *create* a joke? The answer lies in the fact that joke-technique diverts attention away from reproach (1905a, p. 52).

Let us take as an example a "logical" joke that uses the technique of displacement to create its jokiness. This is a Jewish "schnorrer" joke that runs as follows:

> An impoverished individual borrowed 25 florins from a prosperous acquaintance, with many assertions of his necessitous circumstances. The very same day his benefactor met him again in a restaurant with a plate of salmon mayonnaise in front of him. The benefactor reproached him: "What? You borrow money from me and then order yourself salmon mayonnaise? Is *that* what you used my money for?" "I don't understand you", replied the object of the attack; "if I haven't any money then I *can't* eat salmon mayonnaise, and if I have some money I *mustn't* eat salmon mayonnaise? Well, then, when *am* I to eat salmon mayonnaise?" (1905a, pp. 49–50)

In this joke, the man replies with an appearance of logic to the reproach as if it had been that he ought not eat salmon mayonnaise *on the same day* that he borrowed money. The reproach, of course, is that he ought not have been thinking of salmon mayonnaise *at all*. "The improverished bon vivant disregards this only possible meaning of the reproach and answers another question as if he had misunderstood the reproach" (p. 50). The technique of displacement diverts attention from the main reproach; it also substitutes a petty reproach on the part of the benefactor, as if it had been his (foolish) meaning. With reproach displaced, and the reproacher made foolish, laughter at the benefactor and at being a "schnorrer" replaces humiliation.

In analyzing nonsensical and absurd jokes, as well as jokes that depend on "unification" of ideas, Freud shows us how the joke-technique diverts attention away from humiliation by turning the tables on the mighty, but in laughter rather than in insult. Thus, for instance, the following example:

> Serenissimus (a royal personage) was making a tour through his provinces and noticed a man who bore a striking resemblance to his own exalted person. He beckoned to him and asked: "Was your mother at one time in service in the Palace'—'No, your Highness, was the reply, "but my father was." (pp. 68–69)

Here is an example of a joke written by Heine, that relies on analogy for its effect:

> A Catholic cleric behaves rather like a clerk with a post in a large business house. The Church, the big firm, of which the Pope is the head, gives him a fixed job and, in return, a fixed salary. He works lazily as everyone does who

is not working for his own profit, who has numerous colleagues and can easily escape notice in the bustle of a large concern. All he has at heart is the credit of the house and still more its maintenance, since if it should go bankrupt he would lose his livelihood. A Protestant cleric, on the other hand, is in every case his own principal and carries on the business of religion for his own profit. He does not, like his Catholic fellow-traders, carry on a wholesale business but only retail. And since he must manage it alone, he cannot be lazy. He must advertise his article of faith, he must depreciate his competitors' articles, and genuine retailer that he is, he stands in his retail shop, full of business envy of all the great houses, and particularly of the great house in Rome, which pays the wages of so many thousands of book-keepers and packers and has its factories in all four quarters of the globe. (p. 87)

The effect of this joke is to render absurd both Catholic and Protes-tant established religion. Clearly, however, the joke cannot have its effect unless the listeners at least were able to hear a voice critical of religion. This joke clearly depends on the empathic relationship be-tween joker and listener. The joke also clearly uses analogy to make both institutions absurd; here the line between laughter and insult is quite unclear.

FREUD'S THEORY OF JOKES

After many examples of different kinds of jokes, Freud addresses the central question: What is the purpose of jokes? He begins by dis-tinguishing between tendentious and nontendentious, or "innocent," jokes. (He remarks that Fischer, a contemporary psychologist, calls these innocent jokes "abstract"; here Freud clearly prefers the more affective term.)

Freud's use of the term "tendentious" (*tendenziös*) clearly specifies that the joke arises in an argument. Webster's dictionary defines "tend-entious" as "marked by an intended reformatory intent, or by an im-plicit purpose or disposition to promote a point of view." From the examples Freud analyzes it is clear that the tendentiousness arises in coping either with a reproach, or with a direct humiliation—that is, it arises out of the hostility evoked in defending the self against either guilt or shame (or both). But, as we have so often seen before, Freud does not explicitly name these affective-cognitive states when he comes to ex-pounding theory. Both the book on mistakes and the book on jokes were, of course, written long before Freud began to conceptualize the superego in its own terms.

Even after he had formulated the concept of superego, however,

Freud still had not distinguished formally between the ego and the self. He had not, in consequence, distinguished formally between shame and guilt. One result is that the way in which one can soften humiliation by laughing at oneself is conceptualized by Freud as the "triumph of narcissism," instead of as the maintenance of attachment. Thus he tells us (1927a) that humor has "something of grandeur and elevation" that results from the "triumph of narcissism, the victorious assertion of the ego's invulnerability" (p. 162). What happens when humor is evoked is that the person "suddenly hypercathects his own superego" and treats his own ego as if it were something "worth making a jest about" (pp. 165–166). The context in which Freud is thinking here is that of danger of actual annihilation. The intention that humor serves is: " 'Look, here is the world which seems so dangerous! It is nothing but a game for children—just worth making a jest about!' " (p. 166). The danger to which Freud is alluding, however, is really not the danger of the actual annihilation of the person (ego) but the momentary danger of the self's temporary annihilation in shame or humiliation vis-à-vis the "other." Humor says: "Don't take yourself so seriously." As Freud himself points out, the superego is also trying to "console the ego and protect it from suffering," a function that "does not contradict its origin in the parental agency" (p. 166). Here, in other words, he is speaking of the superego not as the punishing internalized agency but as the comforting agency, a distillation of positive attachment feelings. Schafer (1960) and Turiel (1967) have both called attention to the neglect of the benign superego in Freudian theory, and I have connected this neglect with the corresponding neglect of shame in psychoanalytic theory (Lewis, 1971).

The awkwardness of Freud's theoretical position is particularly clear when one reviews his account of obscene jokes, which are smut transformed into a joking version. The model Freud uses for both smut and obscene jokes is the oedipal triangle within which exhibitionism and scopophilia have been evoked by the woman's refusal of a man's wooing.

> Generally speaking, a tendentious joke calls for three people: in addition to the one who makes the joke, there must be a second who is taken as the object of the hostility or sexual aggressiveness and a third in whom the joke's aim of producing pleasure is fulfilled. . . . when the first person finds his libidinal impulses inhibited by the woman, he develops a hostile trend against that ally. Through the first person's smutty speech the woman is exposed before the third who, as listener, has now been bribed by the effortless satisfaction of his own libido. (1905a, p. 100)

Undisguised, smut, which is a direct source of laughter in uneducated peasant society, is unacceptable among more refined persons. "We . . .

could never bring ourselves to laugh at the coarse smut, we should feel ashamed or it would seem to us disgusting. We can only laugh when a joke has come to our help" (p. 101).

The main point of this exposition is that jokes function to connect in shared laughter persons who might otherwise be in a shared state of guilt or humiliation. But in the very same pages in which Freud is conceptualizing this account of a complicated social interaction, he relies only on the "satisfaction of an instinct" as his base.

> At last we can understand what it is that jokes achieve in the service of their purpose. They make possible the satisfaction of an instinct (whether lustful or hostile) in the face of an obstacle that stands in its way. They circumvent this obstacle and in that way draw pleasure from a source which the obstacle had made inaccessible. The obstacle standing in the way is in reality nothing other than women's incapacity to tolerate undisguised sexuality, an incapacity correspondingly increased with a rise in the educational and social level. . . . The power which makes it difficult or impossible for women, and to a lesser degree for men as well, to enjoy undisguised obscenity is termed by us "repression." (pp. 100–101)

In this theoretical account, jokes function to release the sexual instinct only.

The reader will have noted that, once again, Freud is in an androcentric position. The woman is the inhibitor of sex; she is by implication more subject to the power of repression. In Freud's view this characteristic, as we saw in Chapter 5, is not the result of her higher moral development, but of the lesser strength of her sexual instinct.

Freud analyzed four categories of jokes: obscene, hostile, cynical, and skeptical. The obscene have just been discussed. His descriptive account of hostile jokes also requires a third person who joins against a common enemy.

> Since we have been obliged to renounce the expression of hostility by deeds—held back by the passionless third person, in whose interest it is that personal security shall be preserved—we have, just as in the case of sexual aggressiveness, developed a new technique by invective, which aims at enlisting this third person against our enemy. By making our enemy small, inferior, despicable or comic, we achieve in a roundabout way the enjoyment of overcoming him—to which the third person, who has made no efforts, bears witness by his laughter. (p. 103)

Tendentious jokes, Freud continues, are "highly suitable for attacks on the great, the dignified and the mighty" (p. 105). They function, in other words, to relieve the humiliation of the lowly by effecting the humiliation of the mighty. How this process of social leveling works, and why it is needed in the first place, are still unsolved problems that

Freud's formulation of the joke as instinct-releaser simply did not address.

Freud's interpretation of cynical jokes is that they are disguised—but very effective and understandable—attacks on the societal institutions of morality and religion.

> What these jokes whisper may be said aloud: that the wishes and desires of men have a right to make themselves acceptable alongside of exacting and ruthless morality. And in our days it has been said in forceful and stirring sentences that this morality is only a selfish regulation laid down by the few who are rich and powerful and who can satisfy their wishes at any time without any postponement. So long as the art of healing has not gone further in making our life safe and so long as social arrangements do no more to make it enjoyable, so long will it be impossible to stifle the voice within us that rebels against the demands of morality. Every honest man will end by making this admission, at least to himself. The decision in this conflict can only be reached through the roundabout path of fresh insight. One must bind one's own life to that of others so closely and be able to identify with others so intimately that the brevity of one's own life can be overcome; and one must not fulfill the demands of one's own need illegitimately, but must leave them unfulfilled, because only the continuance of so many unfulfilled demands can develop the power to change the order of society. But not every personal need can be postponed in this way and transferred to other people, and there is no general and final solution to the conflict. (1905a, p. 110)

Freud sympathizes with both sides—with the critic of hypocritical and oppressive morality, and with the necessity for a morality that binds people together. It is a cynical *joke* that can express both sides of feeling in congruent thoughts that are immediately comprehensible.

Here is Freud's example of a witty cynical joke: "A wife is like an umbrella—sooner or later one takes a cab" (p. 110). The simile between wife and umbrella is perfectly congruent with the meaning of taking a wife as a protection; the allusion to taking a cab as taking a public facility—or prostitute—also represents a congruence between thought and feeling.

> One does not venture to declare aloud and openly that marriage is not an arrangement calculated to satisfy a man's sexuality, unless one is driven to do so perhaps by the love of truth. . . . The strength of this joke lies in the fact that nevertheless—in all kinds of roundabout ways—it *has* declared (Freud's italics). One might add that, in this instance, the joke has declared on the side of comforting the cynic, who is also clearly a man. (1905a, p.111)

(This is another example of Freud's sexism and of the bias that leads him to neglect his own just-stated defense of renunciation as leading to changes in the social order.)

In his theoretical formulation Freud did not consider the uniqueness of the phenomena of jokes, but was more concerned to show similarities between the "joke work" and primary process in dreams and symptoms. Faced with explaining how a momentary lapse of attention can instigate the complicated intellectual operations that issue in a joke, Freud used the same concept of the unconscious as a storehouse of emotionally charged symbols that he invoked for dreams. The emphasis in this theoretical line is on the power of the unconscious as synonymous with the power of the emotions. The emotions that so powerfully divert attention away from themselves are the "negative" or painful ones—shame and guilt. That both of these states themselves press toward the restoration of positive affectional ties is overlooked, or else this concept is expressed in the notion of "undischarged" cathexis. Nowhere is it clearer, however, than in the uniquely social nature of jokes—which collapse when the joker and listener are not in accord—that this aspect of human functioning was short-changed in Freud's metapsychology.

The general neglect of Freud's work on jokes has also resulted in a neglect of his descriptions of the *congruence* between cognition and affect. Also neglected is Freud's reliance on such cognitive "laws" as "sense in nonsense," "bewilderment and illumination," and "unification of ideas." In Freud's metapsychology the central concept became that affects *distort* cognitions, as they often do in mistakes, dreams, and symptoms. Primary process took on a general meaning of "primitive," as opposed to higher-level cognitive functioning; affects became synonymous with disorganization.

The issues raised by Freud's work on jokes have remained more or less outside the mainstream of both psychoanalysis and academic psychology. That mental patients are not free to appreciate humor is an accepted clinical observation in keeping with Freud's description of jokes, but the dynamics of that phenomenon have only rarely been explored (Levine, 1979). This is another reflection of the discrepancy between Freud's clinical description of neurosis as a transformation of undischarged shame and guilt, and his theoretical account.

FREUD'S THEORY OF "PRIMARY PROCESS"

Nowhere is the absence of a viable theory of human emotional connectedness more apparent than in Freud's theoretical account of the "primary process," the process by which affects influence cognitions.

In order to look very closely at Freud's theoretical position we need to consult again Chapter 7 of his *Interpretation of Dreams*, the principal place in which he put forth his concept of the primary and secondary processes. This theoretical account came to include everyday psycho-pathology and jokes as well, although it was originally written for dreams. It is fascinating to consider how close Freud came to having a social theory of human nature and human emotions, since the examples on which he bases his model have to do with the infant and its caretaker. Freud's theory directly involves the *absent* caretaker in the genesis of emotions; it is when the caretaker is present that the result is an "experi-ence of satisfaction" that is essentially "perception." Had his model allowed for the direct evocation of positive affect in the caretaker's pres-ence, his system could have been a "social" one. (To be sure, the results of the Harlows' work on mothering were not yet available.)

Here is Freud's "schematic picture of the psychical apparatus."

> Hypotheses, whose justifications must be looked for in other directions, tell us that at first the apparatus's efforts were directed toward keeping itself so far as possible free from stimuli; consequently its first structure followed the plan of a reflex apparatus, so that any sensory excitation impinging on it could be promptly discharged along a motor path. But the exigencies of life interfere with this simple function, and it is to this, too, that the apparatus owes the impetus to further development. The exigencies of life confront it first in the form of the major somatic needs. The excitations produced by internal needs seek discharge in movement, which may be described as an "internal change" or an *"expression of emotion"* [italics added]. A hungry baby screams or kicks helplessly. But the situation remains unaltered, for the excitation arising from an internal need is not due to a force producing a momentary impact but to one which is in continuous operation. A change can come about if in some way or other (in the case of the baby, through *outside* help) [italics added] an "experience of satisfaction" can be achieved which puts an end to the internal stimulus. An essential component of this experience of satisfaction is a particular perception (that of nourishment, in our example) the mnemic image of which remains associated thenceforward with the memory trace of the excitation produced by the need. As a result of the link that has thus been established, next time this need arises a psychical impulse will at once emerge which will seek to recathect the mnemic image of the perception and to reevoke the perception itself, that is to say, to re-establish the situation of the original satisfaction. An impulse of this kind is what we call a wish. (1900, pp. 565–566)

What Freud is saying in this account is that emotions are by-prod-ucts of instinctual frustrations. The emphasis is on the absent "object" and the resulting negative affects of protest. When it comes to the "ex-perience and satisfaction" of the need, Freud does not appear to be speaking of affects, directly evoked, but of perceptions and memory traces of the nourishment obtained by means of which the "experience of satisfaction" is learned. This is a framework in which the "internal" excitations produced by instincts are differentiated from the "external" stimuli coming from the "nourishment." What this formulation omits is the existence of positive affects accompanying the mere presence of the "object," or in modern formulation, the positive attachment-emotions that seem to lubricate rather than disrupt the reflex arc.

As we have seen in Chapter 5, Freud conceptualized affects according to Darwin's model as inherited instinctive responses guaranteeing species survival. The emphasis in Darwin's formulation was on the dangers of food scarcity and of predation—what present-day ethologists would call the agonic mode of social organization under threat. Newer information suggests that a theoretical model must also accommodate the affects arising in the hedonic or peaceful mode of social organization (Chance, 1980).

It is fascinating to speculate (with hindsight) on how Freudian theory might have been formulated had the adaptive exigencies of the nurturant mother and her infant been conceptualized as a guiding principle of evolution. If smooth emotional bonding is the focal concept, then cognition is assumed to work in order to maintain it, and also to work best when it is operating within emotional bonding. Studies of human infant sociability can readily be accommodated to a new, yet thoroughly Freudian framework in which positive as well as negative affects are included as basic to all human functioning.

Several consequences follow from Freud's use of the agonic mode of social organization. The affects of fear, want, and threat take first place as the basic inherited adaptive responses. *All* affects are then seen as arising out of threat to individual survival. The affects on which the model focuses are, however, the "negative" affects—those that are often disorganizing to the smooth functioning of the individual's behavior. This is an emphasis from which one can slip easily into the hypothesis that all affects are inherently disorganizing or "primitive," and that the task of the developing human being is to change affects into "cognitive signals."

Still another chain of theorizing is set in motion by a model that starts from the disorganizing negative affects. Because the threatened aggressions in the model imply real dangers, the cognitions that accompany the negative affects are understood as valid representations of real-world events, including those arising "within" the organism, as, for instance, hunger. But if the cognitive representations are valid and the negative affects (by implication) "appropriate," how do these veridical cognitions and appropriate affects arise out of disorganization? A tortuous question then arises—one that also plagued Freud (1926): What is the primary force in the development of valid cognition? Negative affect?

Two theoretical models were developed within the Freudian system to answer these questions. In one theoretical model—Freud's own (1900, 1926), more fully expounded by Anna Freud (1946)—all cognitions originate in the negative affect associated with physical danger. Here is Anna Freud's official version of Freudian theory:

> If within the id a state of calm and satisfaction prevails, so that there is no occasion for any instinctual impulse to invade the ego in search of gratification and there to produce feelings of tension and "pain," we can learn nothing of the id-contents. It follows, at least theoretically, that the id is not under all conditions open to observation. (p. 5)

In this theoretical statement emotions are basic to life (they are instincts), but only the negative ones are open to observation. By implication, the positive emotions are unknowable.

A second psychoanalytic model was developed by Hartmann (1951) to correct the concept that all cognitions are born out of negative affect. Hartmann's "conflict-free" ego-sphere was a compromise position, which proposed that some veridical cognitions arise in direct adaptive response to what Hartmann specified as the "average expectable environment." Had Hartmann's formulation explicitly specified an average expectable *benign* environment, that addition would have made it possible to retain Freud's major thesis that all cognitions derive from affects. As it was formulated, however, Hartmann's correction continues to assume the individualistic nature of the organism, and a dichotomy between affect and cognition. It assumes, also, that affect influences cognition only if it is "negative," and it thus by implication equates affect with "disturbances" of cognition.

Hartmann's correction also leaves intact that aspect of Freud's theoretical view of the relation between affect and cognition in which the former is specified as primitive and the latter as an advanced form of human behavior. Rapaport's (1960) effort to systematize psychoanalytic theory by distinguishing between a special clinical theory and a general theory of human behavior rests on this emphasis in Hartmann. In fact, Rapaport, following Hartmann, specifically equates primary-process and secondary-process modes of functioning with primitive and more advanced thinking, respectively. Yet in Freud's descriptions of clinical phenomena, whether symptom, dream content, everyday mistakes, or jokes, it is clear that primary-process transformations are not primitive but often very sophisticated ways in which thought symbolizes feeling and vice versa. This line of thinking has since found clear expression in the work of Sharpe (1949) on the dream as metaphor, and in the work of Kris (1952) and Levine (1979), who have pursued the elegant workings of primary process in artistic creation and in the psychology of humor.

Another consequence of the primacy of negative affects is the development of a confusing distinction between internal and external stimuli. In Freud's system negative affects are internally generated from somatic sources, whereas positive affects are learned by association with the "external" source of relief from frustration. That is what Bowlby has called the "cupboard-love theory" of human attachment emotions, since it makes positive social feeling a secondary derivative of frustration.

Still another consequence of the primacy of negative affects is the inviting hierarchical comparison it suggests between lofty reason and disorganizing emotion. As we saw earlier in this chapter, the instances in which Freud, in his theoretical account, changed an affective description of clinical events into a cognitive version are particularly striking in *The Psychopathology of Everyday Life* (1901b), as well as in the theoretical version he used of this material in his later writings.

A model of the relation between affect and cognition formed along the lines suggested by hedonic social organization has yet to be fully developed. But it is clear that positive affects of interest, satisfaction, pleasure, and joy also arise in veridical cognition of a nonthreatening environment—that is, one of a friendly, affectionate interaction between the organism and its caretaker. In any case, there is no intrinsic reason why both positive and negative emotions may not be associated with need gratification and frustration through the relationship with the caretaker. The association between emotion and frustration alone is a product of an individualistic theory of human nature under threat, which then has difficulty incorporating the role of positive experiences with the "other."

There have been some recent attempts to find a bridge between Freudian theory and present-day information-processing theories of cognition (Erdelyi, 1974; Bowlby, 1980). These efforts are based on the similarity between Freud's concept of "overload" (i.e., the tendency to keep the organism free of stimulus buildup) and the assumption in cognitive theory that the cognitive system is limited in the amount of information it can process. Erdelyi (1974) reminds us that there is "no truer truism in contemporary cognitive psychology" (p. 20) than the idea that the system must be selective. In addition to an intrinsic limitation in scope (with which neither Freudian observation nor information-processing theory has any quarrel), Freud's observations led him to the theory that negative emotions are the factor governing overload. In order to develop this hypothesis he had to oppose it to the prevailing doctrine of his time. Both Charcot and Janet believed that it was some "psychic insufficiency," or cognitive defect, that led to the splitting of consciousness or stimulus overload. Freud, in contrast, insisted that the splitting of consciousness was itself the result of an "act of will on the part of the patient" (1894, p. 46). This act of will was the result of an

> incompatibility of their ideational life . . . their ego was faced with an experience, an idea or a feeling which aroused such a distressing affect that the subject decided to forget about it because he had no confidence in his power to resolve the contradiction between that incompatible idea and his ego by means of thought-activity. (p. 47)

Freud thus located the basis of selectivity in the avoidance of distressing affect (without, as we have seen so often, specifying the distressing affects as guilt and shame). In his theoretical formulations he also focused on the concept of overload: "The mental apparatus endeavours to keep the quantity of excitation present in it as low as possible or at least to keep it constant" (1920, p. 9). In Freud's metapsychology, undischarged (negative) emotions are specifically regarded as the cause of the overload, or as the locus of bias in determining what enters the (information-processing) system. Sometimes the excessive (affective) stimulation comes "from without," as in the case of traumatic (terrifying) events on the battlefield, but most often the excessive stimulation comes from the "instincts." (This is another example of the confusing meaning of a stimulus "from without." Here the "outside stimulus" is not the nurturant mother but the imminent threat of death.) The "instincts" produce a "quota of affect" or a "sum of excitations" that makes the system necessarily selective for fear of overload. The results of the selection are one or another form of cognitive distortion, either total ideational blackout, as in denial or somatic conversion, or a discrepancy between affective and cognitive content, as in the isolation of affect in obsessional neurosis and paranoia.

Thus Freud's concept of overload entails two corollaries. One is that affects are the inherent causes of overload: They are thus inherently disorganizing in their effect. Logic, however, does not require this characteristic of affect. On the contrary, positive affects can function as silent facilitators of cognitive operations, or they can also create overload. The second corollary is that there is a "normal" cognitive processing system (secondary process) that operates smoothly when there are *no* affects. (This is the place where most information-processing theories start.) But this proposition is also not necessary—if we have learned anything over the past several decades it is that the benign affects of interest and attention, as well as positive self-regard, are a necessary but not sufficient condition for smooth cognitive functioning. Many of the laws of "cognitive" psychology so skillfully assembled by experimental psychologists are obtained from subjects whose quiet, good-humored cooperation during the experiment is taken for granted.

Bowlby (1980) has recently attempted to form a bridge between information-processing theory and the psychoanalytic concepts of defense. He postulates that a "principal [information-processing] system" consists of "one or more principal evaluators and controllers closely linked to long-term memory and comprising a very large number of evaluation [appraisal] scales ranged in some order of precedence" (p. 52). It should be noted that Bowlby has avoided the dichotomy between affect and cognition by simply assuming the existence of "evaluators" or "appraisers" as a "given." The union of affect and cognition is thus assumed *a priori* in the process of evaluative selection. Although Bowlby does not explicitly make a connection between his model of an information-processing system and his own work on attachment, it seems feasible to connect the power of the affective ties that govern human behavior with the "limited capacity" of an information-processing system. The (limited) information-processing system selects preferentially what is relevant to the maintenance of (powerful) affective ties.

Recently two separate developments, both calling themselves "script theory" (Abelson, 1981; Tomkins, 1980), have addressed the age-old problem of the relation between cognition and affect. Both these theories emphasize the congruity or coherence between cognition and affect. Abelson's script theory appears to have come into being out of criticism of cognitive psychology for being overly elementaristic and for ignoring the dynamic natural cognitive processes (Abelson, 1976) that characterize some computer simulation models of information processing. Tomkins's script theory comes out of an effort to flesh out the cognitive side of his theory that affects, the "amplifiers" of behavior, are fundamental to motivation. Tomkins's theory conceptualizes the person as the "playwright" or organizer of his/her experiences into "nuclear scenes," encoded in long-term memory and forming a script for the interpretation of present experience. Abelson's scripts are broad-ranging and describe such varied phenomena as expectancy-sets in everyday routine experiences, and in such feelings as anger, pride, or guilt. Abelson recognizes that feelings are "conceptually very coherent" (1981, p. 727). The script that describes anger at injustice includes blaming and punishing the unjust aggressor, as well as swearing and excitement, in a coherent cognitive and affective whole.

Abelson's script theory has been used as a guide to the experimental study of behavior in a way that illustrates the usefulness of assuming a coherence between cognition and affect, rather than a dichotomy. One example is Langer and Abelson's (1972) study of the semantics of asking a favor. They compared two common scripts that could be used in asking for help: an *empathy* script, emphasizing a victim's hurt, and a more straightforward *social obligation* script. Langer and Abelson predicted that the *legitimacy* of the help asked for by the victim would be a much more powerful determinant in the empathy script than in the social obligation script. An illegitimate request in the empathy script would "interrupt" it and make the victim not worth one's sympathy. As predicted, the legitimacy of the favor asked made a much greater difference to the frequency of helping in the empathy script than it did in the social obligation script.

Psychoanalysis would have little difficulty in agreeing with Langer and Abelson's scripts for the power of legitimacy to structure a situation in which empathy for another human being is evoked. Some might consider the script as a reflection of how closeness to others "naturally" sharpens disappointment at betrayal and increases subsequent vigilance. But whatever language is used to describe a complicated affective and cognitive interaction, a congruence between empathy (an *affective*-cognitive state) and legitimacy (a *cognitive*-affective state) is implied. (it is *good* to help a victim when it is *really* needed. It is *foolish* to help a victim when he/she is *inappropriately* demanding.) In any case, the appearance of such scripts in the thinking of academic psychologists suggests that the vexed problem of the relation between affect and cognition with which Freud struggled is being studied anew with an awareness of the complexity of the relationship that he was the first to describe.

CHAPTER 7

Psychoanalytic Characterology
The Problem of Cognitive Styles

Freud's major observations on cognitive styles, in addition to those in his work on unraveling symptoms, dreams, mistakes, and jokes, are found in three of his "minor" writings. The first source is Freud's early description of the differences among the defenses of conversion, isolation of affect, and total repression (Freud, 1894, 1896), a distinction still being studied between "repressors" and "sensitizers" (Byrne, 1964), or between people with "high and low vigilance" (Minard, 1965). The second source is Freud's description of the anal character (1908a), another kind of statement of cognitive style, this time based on a theory of moral development. It is this paper that was the model for an extrapolated "oral" character. The third source is Freud's description of masculine and feminine cognitive styles, based on the interaction between sex and culturally prescribed sex roles and culminating in a sex difference in style of conscience, that is, in the relationship between the self and internalized others. These concepts found brief expression in Freud's paper on libidinal types (1931), and have been picked up in the work on field dependence, as well as in studies on locus of control (Rotter, 1966). The present chapter will review these three sources, and will trace the ways in which they have influenced the mainstream of psychology.

Reviewing these three sources will demonstrate how profound Freud's influence has been in both "state" and "trait" psychology of personality. His concepts have permeated the climate of observation about personality in a way so taken for granted that "new" evidence arises without awareness of its source in Freudian thinking. A recent example is the rapidly growing body of work on Type A personality and coronary disease. The evolution of this description of the "driven" man out of Freud's (1908a) anal character as revised into Fromm's (1941) "bourgeois" character has apparently been lost in the depths of psychology's "unconscious" (or in its apperceptive mass, depending upon how "cognitive" or "dynamic" one's view). To most of the present generation of psychologists the two cardiologists who observed the personalities of coronary patients appeared to be making entirely new observations, instead of observations already embedded not only in the Freudian concept of "psychosomatics" but also in the popular absorption of the concept of bourgeois character into the concept of an "organization man."

An awareness of the historical roots of concepts is not only a good thing in its own right, it can help to pinpoint problems that were apparent at the time of formulation and still exist. For example, as might have been predicted from Freudian thinking, the applicability of the Type A characterization to women is one still unsolved major problem (Waldron, 1978). There is an association between Type A personality and coronary disease in women, as there is in men. But women, in general, score lower than men on the Type A scale, and their position in the hierarchy of corporate power is lower, as is their death rate from coronary disease. The problem that thus emerges is the same as Freud faced: Is there something genetic in women's lower death rate in addition to the obvious difference in life style and socialization?

Another problem predictable from Freudian thinking is the role of sociability in the relation between Type A personality and coronary disease. Recent work on Type A men (Jenkins, Zyzanski, Ryan, Flessas, & Tannenbaum, 1977) has shown that their driven, competitive behavior is accompanied also by social awkwardness and discomfort when in groups. Both competitiveness and social awkwardness predict coronary disease. Is it competitiveness or is it social awkwardness that is the main contributor? Or do these two factors necessarily involve each other? If one assumes that human beings are social (sexual, in Freud's thinking) by nature, then one may suppose that men pay a high price for their competitiveness in the antisocial demands it makes upon them (and physical demands on their hearts).

THE NEUROPSYCHOSIS OF DEFENSE: REPRESSION VERSUS
ISOLATION OF AFFECT

A rereading of Freud's seminal papers on the differences between
conversion and isolation of affect highlights the problems he raised that
are still unsolved. It is also helpful to trace the subtle but important
changes that took place in his exposition as he moved further away from
his own direct clinical observations into speculations. This is particularly
significant for the fate of the concept of "conversion," which Freud first
described in women hysterical patients. Even though his first clinical
description of what happens clearly suggests that *both* idea and affect are
"weakened" consciously and *not* totally lost to awareness, Freud's later
metapsychological paper on repression (1915b) suggests that conversion
is preceded by total cognitive loss. By this time in his writings, total
cognitive loss was also considered a greater psychological deficit than
the distortions imposed by obsessive ideas. Thus the *"belle indifference"*
of hysterical women was once again a source of covert ridicule of wom-
en's apparent inability to understand their own transparent symptoms.
By a similar process, repression came to be considered a simpler or more
primitive defense than isolation of affect (the more frequent cognitive
style of male obsessionals).

What initiates a defense in Freud's earliest version is the occurrence
of an "incompatibility . . . in ideational life" (1894, p. 47). (As discussed
in Volume 1, Freud apparently used the terms "incompatible" and "unbearable" interchangeably, even though the latter is much more affectively laden than the former). As we have seen so often already, the
"incompatibility" to which Freud refers is actually the affective state of
guilt and/or shame. Here are two of his examples of how patients form
the intention of "pushing the thing away" (the incompatibility):

> The case of a girl who *blamed* herself because, while she was nursing her sick
> father she thought about a young man who had made a slight erotic impres-
> sion on her; the case of a governess who had fallen in love with her employer
> and had resolved to drive this inclination out of her mind because it seemed
> to her incompatible with her *pride;* and so on. (p. 48, italics added)

Freud very cautiously suggests in this first paper that trying to
forget about something unresolvable is not inherently pathological, and
also that some people succeed in doing so and remain healthy. (The
problem of the etiology of neurosis that Freud mentions here is still,
even today, not solved.) In some pathological instances, however, further defense is needed because guilt and shame will not resolve. Then
what happens is that both the idea and the affect are "weakened," not

ablated. Freud reserves the latter description for cases of hallucinatory psychosis. The weakened conscious affect is also detached from its weakened "idea." But the affect (although consciously weakened) still retains the power of its "sum of excitations" that must be discharged. Up to this point hysteria, phobia, and obsessional neurosis share the same process. But in hysteria, the powerful affect is *"transformed into something somatic"* (p. 49, Freud's italics).

For unknown reasons, "people who lack the aptitude for conversion" (p. 51) set about separating the incompatible idea from its affect. (The problem of individual differences in "choice" of defense is still not solved.) The affect remains fully conscious, but it is attached to other ideas, not in themselves incompatible, but clearly "false connections" in the cognitive systems of the patient himself. Thus the patient *knows* that he/she is not guilty but nevertheless is tortured by the obsessive idea that he is. Similarly, the patient knows that he is not afraid—that there is really no reason to be afraid—but is tortured by the realization that he feels afraid in spite of his reason.

Both somatic conversion and displacement of affect onto "false connections" are frankly hypothetical processes designed to fill the "gap" that "yawns" (P. (p. 53) between the patient's effort of will in "weakening" unacceptable sexual ideas and the emergence of symptoms. It should be noted that the hypothetical status of defensive processes was acknowledged again in the 1915 papers on metapsychology. In both papers, Freud's attention was focused on the intervening steps between cognitive weakening and symptom formation. It was already clear that many different kinds of defensive maneuvers were involved, including reaction formation, that is, the development of "conscientiousness," regression to earlier developmental stages (mainly anal), and undoing (of the guilty act). Clearly these additional defensive maneuvers were designed to explain the steps involved in obsessional ideas rather than in the formation of somatic symptoms. Freud's attention in the papers on metapsychology is focused on the cognitive side of the defensive maneuvers—on what remains conscious and what evades awareness—rather than on the relation of the self to the significant "other."

In his later speculations, as well as in the first clinical description, Freud clearly regards ideas as more susceptible to ablation than affects, which are (after all) the "charged" representatives of instincts seeking discharge. It is the unquenchable affects that keep pushing ideas down out of awareness and pushing them up into awareness. In his paper on the unconscious, for example, Freud insists that "to suppress the development of affect is the true aim of repression" (1915b, p. 178). From this point of view, the conversion of affect directly into somatic symptoms leaves the "ego" (self) relatively unscathed, whereas the persistence of obsessive ideas that accompanies detachment or isolation of affect is the source of persistent ego disturbance. This early contrast in cognitive style has since been generally reversed to favor the more "sophisticated" obsessional defenses as more advanced developmentally (see Volume 1). This could have been predicted from Freud's emphasis on the value of ideas in contrast to the affects, which are only primitive instinct representatives however powerful. Once again, as we saw in Chapter 6, the (negative) affects are conceived of as powerful but primitive; "secondary" processes, which only barely contain them, are nevertheless rational and thus of a higher order.

A reformulation that starts with states of unresolvable guilt and shame as the instigators of "defense," and supposes that these states operate so as to keep the person attached to significant others, permits the notion that ideas and affects work congruently toward the maintenance of attachment. (Neither idea nor affect is of a higher order.) When a guilt–shame state is succeeded by a somatic illness, the person is now blameless, although distressingly helpless physically, needing another's intervention. There is, moreover, the actual likelihood that whatever autonomic arousal has been involved in a chronic shame/guilt state can directly evoke somatic changes. When the same (unresolvable) guilt/shame state is followed by the outbreak of worrisome or "guilty" ideas that make no rational sense, the person is clearly unable to find a stance that keeps him/her peacefully attached to significant others. In part this is a function of the ideational quality of guilt itself, which can alternatively blame and exonerate (mainly by blaming the other), and which gives "isolation of affect" its apparent hierarchical placement as developmentally more advanced.

CHARACTER AND ANAL-EROTISM

The most important paper in which Freud opened up the question of cognitive style was that in which he described the anal-erotic character (1908a). The impression of a connection between adult character and childhood anality came unexpectedly to Freud: "I can assure the reader that no theoretical expectation played a part in that impression . . . the intrinsic necessity for this connection was not clear" to Freud (pp. 169, 172). Freud speculated, however, that the emotions stirred during toilet training are still operative in the form of a triad of adult character traits. Two distinct hypotheses are implied in his paper: the existence of a triad of adult traits; and the origin of this triad in a "sublimation" of childhood anal-erotism. This second hypothesis assumes that morality itself develops as a sublimation of "the excitations proceeding from the erotogenic zones" (p. 171), and that anal-erotism is the specific component out of which the adult triad is transformed. A psychoanalytic characterology is thus specifically based in a morality that is theoretically derived from the sexual instinct. Or, as it is put in one modern-day version (Lewis, 1976), psychoanalytic characterology is based on morality, which itself evolves out of the social nature of the human self.

Let us look more closely at the first part of Freud's hypothesis—the existence of the adult character triad. Freud's description clearly uses each of three words to cover

> a small group of interrelated character-traits. "Orderly" covers the notion of bodily cleanliness, as well as of conscientiousness in carrying out small duties and trustworthiness. Its opposite would be "untidy" and "neglectful". Parsimony may appear in the exaggerated form of avarice; and obstinacy can go over into defiance, to which rage and revengefulness are easily joined. The two latter qualities—parsimony and obstinacy—are linked with each other more closely than they are with the first—with orderliness. They are, also, the more constant element of the whole complex. Yet it seems to me incontestable that all three in some way belong together. (p. 169)

Each of these classes of traits clearly involves a style of cognition, as well as of affective attitudes. Each of the classes can also have a very different value put on it, depending on the context in which the trait is being evaluated, or on the observer's point of view. Cleanliness, for example, is a virtue in a hospital surgery room; it is also (since Freud) the mark of a "compulsive housewife" in the eyes of her angry adolescent son. Orderliness itself can be regarded as pedantic and constricted, or else as systematic or even as aesthetically sensitive, depending on the context in which orderliness is being practiced. Conscientiousness in carrying out small duties and trustworthiness, for example, in meeting deadlines or quotas of work—the opposite of neglectful or untidy—are virtues in the business office, or in an agricultural enterprise, in which neglect or failure to meet deadlines can be a disaster. But in other contexts, such conscientiousness can also be regarded as "compulsive" or "driven," the mark of an alienated, emotionally isolated man who cares more about his deadlines than about personal relationships. Parsimony, as Freud says, goes over into avarice; but it can also be a virtue called thrift or planfulness, including an appreciation of the value of money well earned for expenditure of effort. Whether a man is stingy or realistically thrifty depends on the context, one's point of view, or one's feeling toward him. Obstinacy, which can go over to defiance, is similarly either the virtue of persistent self-assertion or courageous aggression, or the person can be irrationally headstrong, ill tempered, and rageful, involving himself in the stress of seeking revenge.

It should be noted that Freud's description of the anal triad developed out of his analysis of obsessional neurotics. The driven quality of obsessive and compulsive thinking, its insistent conscientious orderliness, evolved out of reaction formations against anal-sadism. Freud does not specifically refer to sadism in his 1908 paper, but defecating on others is pleasurably symbolic of their humiliation. Each of the three categories of interrelated traits also clearly involves a style of cognition: orderly-systematic versus loose; parsimonious versus uninterested in money; obstinate versus yielding in one's relations to others. As is apparent even from this brief review of the cognitive and affective implications of each of the traits, the positive and negative values connoted by the triad depend upon the morality of the observer. It is this self-evident variation in evaluation that led Fromm (1941) to recognize Freud's anal triad as a reflection of character traits needed by the capitalist-entrepreneur and deprecated by critics of the profit system. Since then Kardiner (1939) has pursued the "modal personality"—oral or anal (similarly formed out of sublimations)—in nonliterate societies. Before returning to the question of cognitive-affective style as molded by cultural values, let us look at the experimental work that has been done by psychologists on validating Freud's anal triad.

EXPERIMENTAL STUDIES OF THE ANAL TRIAD

Fisher and Greenberg (1977), reviewing 19 empirical studies of the existence of the anal triad, conclude that the studies "have almost unanimously found it possible to isolate recognizable clusters of anal traits and attitudes" (p. 144). One of the most rigorous series of studies replicating Freud's description of the anal triad is Kline's (1971). Kline developed a 30-item self-report measure of the anal triad. Attention was paid in developing the instrument to countering social-desirability and response-set factors. In addition to checking its internal consistency and face validity, Kline was able to check its construct validity. In three separate checks of the construct validity of his measure, Kline showed that it correlated with two separate previously established measures of the anal triad, by Beloff (1957) and Sandler and Hazari (1960).

But perhaps the most striking empirical confirmation of the acuteness of Freud's description of the anal character in adulthood comes from the work on Type A personality. The cardiologists who began some years ago to observe the personalities of men patients who had suffered heart attacks apparently did not relate their observations to Freud's work or to Fromm's (1941), but simply described what they saw: "driven" men. The description of Type A behavior (based on interviews with their coronary patients) made use of such phrases as "excessive drive," "pressure for meeting deadlines." These characteristics are what Freud had in mind when he spoke of orderliness and obstinacy. Type A patients' impatience and competitiveness are another aspect of their obstinacy "going over into" rage and vengefulness. Finally, the Type A patients were, as their investment in their work implies, very much concerned also with the power and prestige that money brings—which evokes a clear reference to Freud's "parsimony." Type B patients, who are less driven than Type A's, are "easy-going," "seldom impatient," and "without a feeling of being driven" (Jenkins, Rosenman, & Friedman, 1967, p. 371). This is something like the oral optimist that Abraham described (see the next two sections). As suggested earlier in this chapter, the work on Type A behavior has opened new ways of studying the sources and consequences of the anal-bourgeois character.

When it comes to an explanation of how the anal triad develops, Freud's hypothesis, although couched in terms of instinctual hydraulics, was also based conceptually on the development of morality. It is in the context of a developed morality that "sublimated" anal-erotism becomes the anal character triad. The "excitations" coming from the erotogenic zones are "deflected from sexual aims and directed toward others—a process that deserved the name of 'sublimation' (1908a, p. 171). Freud actually assumes here, as he does throughout his writings, that morality is rooted in deflected instincts. In this sense, morality is a "given" of human nature in human society. As he puts it:

> Counter-forces, such as shame, disgust and morality are created in the mind. They are actually formed at the expense of the excitations proceeding from the erotogenic zones, and they rise like dams to oppose the later activity of the sexual instincts. (p. 171)

Each of the three adult traits is embedded in a moral context and originates in a complicated process of morality building in childhood. The traits are thus more than residuals or partial instincts. Obstinacy, for example, is the derivative of the child's defiance of his mother who is teaching him how and when to produce his stool. The symbolic connection between money and feces is apparent in shared myths about valued substances. For example, "The gold which the devil gives to his paramours turns to excrement after his departure and the devil is certainly nothing less than the personification of the repressed unconscious instinctual life" (p. 174). Freud further suggests (ibid.) that the contrast between the most precious substance known to men and the most worthless which they reject as waste matter ("refuse") has led to this specific identification of gold with feces. Freud's explanation of the development of the anal character triad thus emphasizes the process of socialization, specifically considering the social interactions that take place around defecation. But his formulation also specifies that anal-erotism is a partial instinct, and it is in keeping with this narrower line of thinking that many experimental studies of the development of the anal character were designed.

Fenichel (1945) set the stage for many studies of the influence of toilet training upon adult character by paraphrasing Freud's concept of an instinct being inhibited:

> The anal-erotic drives meet in infancy with the training for cleanliness, and the way in which this training is carried out determines whether or not anal fixations result. The training may be too early, too late, too strict, too libidinous. (p. 305)

Reviewing the many studies of either extremely lax or extremely strict toilet training in relation to adult anal character, Fisher and Greenberg conclude (1977, p. 146) that there is little support for the extremes-of-toilet-training hypothesis.

But observations independently arrived at by several of the studies suggest a connection between the degree of mother's anality and the child's. Fisher and Greenberg cite these studies as particularly impressive. Beloff (1957) (whose study also affirmed the existence of an anal triad in adulthood) found a significant positive relationship between the degree of anality in men and women college students and the degree of anality (as measured by the same questionnaire) in their mothers. Finney (1963) predicted and confirmed a relationship between a mother's rigidity and her child's anality. That mother's (anal) personality is more potent predictor of her child's anality than her specific toilet-training practices suggests that it is the social interaction between herself and her child that is predictive rather than the extent to which she inhibits or indulges an instinct. As Kline (1971) remarks, this finding is congruent with Fromm's reformulation of Freud's triad.

Fromm's (1941, 1955) reformulation of Freudian characterology has had a far-reaching influence, especially on the development of a psychoanalytic social anthropology, as we shall see in Chapter 9. Fromm's critique of Freud's psychosexual stages rests on a Marxist critique of capitalism's alienating effect on human development. Fromm follows Freud's description of the anal character formation very closely, but he relates the process not only to individual drives and to the family's social interactions, but the the psychological "requirements" of the larger social order. Human adult personality, in this view, is the mortar that holds together the bricks of social institutions (Fromm, 1941). Capitalism's freeing of the individual from the bonds of feudalism also brought with it the individual's isolation, and with it the "insecurity of the isolated individual." It is from this insecurity of aloneness that a person evolves into a competitive, hoarding, exploitative, authoritarian, aggressive and individualistic human being. That is what Fromm calls a nonproductive orientation to the world. Specifically, the (anal) person relates to the world by acquiring things; he assimilates himself to the world by hoarding things and preserving them. Hoarding involves the person in "destructiveness" to others, although it can also evoke "assertiveness." Hoarding also requires a cautious and orderly way of doing things; it can also evoke pedantic and obsessional thinking. Fromm thus expands Freud's theory of the origin of the anal character into a critique of the social order. From this point of view, the evidence accumulating about how Type A behavior kills people, especially men, through its stress on their hearts can be considered striking evidence of the value of psychoanalytic characterology.

THE ORAL CHARACTER

The concept of an oral character in adulthood did not evolve out of a compelling observation of Freud's, as did the anal triad. On the question of the infant's earliest experiences, Freud was caught up in the complexities and obscurities of the first appearance of the sexual instinct, which he located in the infant's experiences at the breast. The sexual nature of sucking at the breast, and of the nonnutritive sucking that also appears in earliest infancy, suggested to Freud that such adult behavior as perverse smoking, drinking, and hysterical vomiting had their origins in oral fixations; but these connections did not amount to a precise description of an adult oral character. The development of a concept of adult oral character was mainly the work of Abraham, Freud's faithful follower, and the concept was much less precise than that of Freud's anal triad.

Before looking at Abraham's model, it is instructive once again to see how prescient Freud was about the importance of nonnutritive sucking. At the same time, Freud's reliance on instinct theory pushed him to an individualistic conception of the suckling infant, thus missing the clearly social nature of nonnutritive sucking. Here is Freud's statement of the sexual basis of sucking and of the child's substitution of a part of his own body for the mother's breast:

To begin with, sexual activity attaches itself to functions *serving the purpose of self-preservation* [italics added] and does not become independent of them until later. No one who has seen a baby sinking back satiated from the breast and falling asleep with flushed cheeks and a blissful smile can escape the reflection that this picture persists as a prototype of the expression of sexual satisfaction in later life. The need for repeating the sexual satisfaction now becomes detached from the need for taking nourishment—a separation which becomes inevitable when teeth appear and food is no longer taken in only by sucking but is also chewed up. The child does not make use of an extraneous body for his sucking, but prefers a part of his own skin because it is more convenient, because it makes him independent of the external world, which he is not yet able to control, and because in that way he provides himself, as it were, with a second erotogenic zone, though one of an inferior kind. The inferiority of this second region is among the reasons why at a later date he seeks the corresponding part—the lips—of another person. ("It's a pity I can't kiss myself," he seems to be saying.) (1905b, p. 182)

The three reasons why the child prefers his own body-part—that it is more convenient, that it makes him "independent," and that it gives him a second, although inferior, erotogenous zone—are all self-evident comparisons between autoerotism and a social-sexual transaction directly involving the mother. What Freud's theory misses, although his description clearly implies it, is that the child learns early to substitute (by simple conditioning, if one is a behaviorist) its own body-part for the missing social transaction. Autoerotic thumbsucking is thus only apparently autistic—it can be an early expression of a conditioned symbolic social-sexual response. Freud need not have got himself into the dilemma implied in assuming that when kissing someone else in later life one is saying "It's a pity I can't kiss myself."

Exactly how nonnutritive sucking in infancy is to be understood is still an open question theoretically, but its existence is not in doubt. Recent 24-hour electroencephalogram monitoring of neonates suggests there are recurring episodes of nonnutritive sucking, in addition to "reflex," apparently nonsocial smiling, startle reactions, and cyclically recurring REM periods (Korner, 1969; Wolff 1969). Theorizing that nonnutritive sucking is part of a socially oriented infant template might be a way of reconciling Freud's "sexual" instinct with the newer evidence of infants' sociability.

In *Three Essays*, Freud, as mentioned earlier, does adumbrate a version of the adult neurotic oral character. He specifically relates a "constitutional intensification" of the "labial region" to adult perverse kissing; smoking and drinking in men; and vomiting in women. In making this kind of connection, Freud assumes that thumb sucking does not occur in every infant, but only in those who are "constitutionally" prone to it. (This assumption, as we have just seen, is contrary to the new evidence that both nonnutritive sucking and thumb sucking are universal.) He writes:

> It is not every child who sucks in this way. It may be assumed that those children do so in whom there is a constitutional intensification of the erotogenic significance to the labial region. If that significance persists, these same children when they are grown up will become epicures in kissing, will be inclined to perverse kissing, or if male, will have a powerful motive for drinking and smoking. If, however, repression ensues, they will feel disgust at food and will produce hysterical vomiting. The repression extends to the nutritive instinct owing to the dual purpose served by the labial zone. Many of my women patients who suffer disturbances of eating, globus hystericus, constriction of the throat and vomiting, have indulged energetically in sucking during their childhood. (p. 182)

Freud's observation of a sex difference in adult addiction to drinking and smoking, as well as in the frequency of anorexia nervosa, is still accurate today, whatever the origin of these symptoms in "orality."

Several important lines of work have issued from Freud's original description of the influences of oral erotogenic zone on later behavior. One line of thinking within the Freudian establishment has been the formulation of an adult affective-cognitive oral style modeled after Freud's concept of "sublimated" anality. Thus Abraham (1924/1965, 1927/1965) developed a version of the adult oral character, and this version, together with additions to it by Glover (1956), has provoked many empirical studies designed to test the model. Another line of development within the psychoanalytic movement has come from the work of Melanie Klein, who translated Freud's theory of eros and the death instinct into a description of infant experience at the "oral" level. In this version of Freudian theory, "object relations" are necessary from the beginning of life to offset the destructive influence of the infant's death instinct. A paranoid, followed by a depressive, position in infant social development sets the stage for later affective-cognitive character styles, including proneness to envy or gratitude. Klein's work is important because it assumes a very early formation of the superego, and because of its influence on Bowlby, who abandoned her theoretical framework but made use of her descriptions of attitude introjections in early infancy. Still another line of development, beginning with Fromm, has attempted to detach Freud's developmental stages from his instinct theory (as we saw in Fromm's translation of the anal character into the bourgeois man). Fromm describes the nonproductive orientation of passivity and wishful thinking that can become oral "receiving"; he also suggests (apparently following Abraham) that optimism and responsiveness develop out of positive oral experiences.

Erikson's (1950) developmental stages, each with its affective-cognitive virtues and dangers, represent still another translation of Freudian partial instincts into social-psychological transactions. In particular, Erikson's first stage, basic trust versus mistrust, closely follows Abraham's oral optimism versus pessimism. It should be noted that Melanie Klein posits an instinctual basis for "object relations," whereas Erikson's position is closer to Hartmann's ego psychology. The reader interested in such details will observe that "object-relations" theory is supposedly a more instinctual or biologically oriented view, in contrast to Fromm, Reich, and Erikson. Ego psychology, however, is equally biological in its assumption that certain cognitive-developmental processes (the "ego-apparatuses") are directly adaptive to the environment, regardless of prevailing "object relations."

Perhaps the most important line of development from the Freudian concept of an adult character formed in intimacy has been the line of experimental work begun by the Harlows, and continuing in the work of Bowlby, Spitz, Mahler, Ainsworth, Sroufe, and many others. Work on the infant–mother social interaction has thus found its way into the mainstream of academic psychology. Its results bear out psychoanalytic predictions that earliest experiences are, indeed, powerful predictors of later cognitive style. Such variables as "self-confidence" and a child's "competence" with its peers are now empirically established as related to the mother–infant interaction; in many instances, these and similar child characteristics are also predictive of adult character.

ABRAHAM'S ORAL CHARACTER

Abraham's (1924/1965) description of the oral character is, as he himself says, disappointing because it does not have nearly the specificity of Freud's anal triad. In part this is because orality "need not be changed into character-formation or sublimated" (p. 394) since its pleasures stay with one throughout life. In fact, the pleasures of sucking are normally simply succeeded by the pleasures of biting, after teeth have erupted: "The child puts every object it can into its mouth and tries . . . to bite it to pieces" (p. 396). Pleasures in sucking and biting at the time of learning and toilet training are then succeeded by the pleasures of retention. Abraham here seems to be describing a peaceful progression of pleasurable stages rather than a series of partial instincts meeting opposition. He is clearly describing a model of pleasurable social experiences in infancy. He adds:

If the pleasure of getting or taking is brought into the most favorable relation possible with the pleasure of possession, as well as with that in giving up, then an exceedingly important step has been made in laying the foundations of the individual's social relations. For when such a relationship between the three tendencies is present, the most important preliminary condition for overcoming the ambivalence of the individual's emotional life has been established. (pp. 396–397)

In this statement, it is emotional ambivalence rather than the nature of the partial instinct that is significant for later development.

Trouble arises when excess occurs in the mother–infant interaction—either indulgence or deprivation. This line of thinking can lend itself to the specifics of frequency and length of time spent either at the breast or in bottle feeding. It can also go beyond such specifics to the broader question of the quality of the mother–infant social interaction. It was actually from the standpoint of the quality of the mother–infant interaction that Abraham made some rather imprecise but nevertheless important and useful observations. So, for example, he notes that "the formation of character of such a child begins under the influence of an abnormally pronounced ambivalence of feeling" (p. 398). Predicting character formation in the light of "undisturbed and highly pleasurable sucking" (p. 399), Abraham writes:

They have brought with them from this happy period of deeply-rooted conviction that everything will always be well with them. They face life with an imperturbable optimism which often does in fact help them to achieve their aims. (p. 399)

"Orally gratified" infants also grow up to be generous, in identification with the "bounteous mother" (p. 403). It is unclear to the reader, however, whether such happy outcomes are the result of unambivalent mother–infant interaction or of excessive oral indulgence.

Abraham goes on, however, to describe a less favorable outcome, this one definitely ascribable to excessive indulgence (and consequent ambivalence of feeling).

Some people are dominated by the belief that there will always be some kind person—a representative of the mother, of course—to care for them and to give them everything they need. This optimistic belief condemns them to inactivity. . . . Their whole attitude towards life shows that they expect the mother's breast to flow for them eternally, as it were. (p. 399)

Finally, Abraham describes the "melancholy seriousness which passes over into marked pessimism" (p. 400) in those people who had to contend with excessive deprivation of their oral needs in infancy.

In persons of this type, the optimistic belief in the benevolence of fate is completely absent. On the contrary, they show an apprehensive attitude towards life, and have a tendency to make the worst of everything and to find undue difficulties in the simplest undertakings. (p. 400)

Both Fisher and Greenberg's (1977) and Kline's (1971) literature reviews of the empirical studies on the oral character agree that the supporting evidence is not strong. Both reviews also agree that the existence of an oral character in adulthood is much less clearly indicated than the anal triad. On the relationship between the adult oral character and infantile oral experience there is even less supporting evidence. In fact, there are contradictory and confusing findings issuing out of the many varieties of experimental probes into this question.

The conceptual difficulties that we have seen in Abraham's formulation seem to me to afford the most likely explanation of why the evidence seems so variable. As one example, the "positive" aspects of orality—that is, imperturbable optimism, generosity, an affiliative and nurturant attitude—are of great use not only in the mother–infant interaction but in later interpersonal relationships. A mother's cheerful patience is often based on her "optimism"; generosity surely helps in many a difficult moment between people. But the values that are placed on such behavior are quite contradictory, depending on the context. Optimism and generosity are not useful characteristics in the aggressive, competitive, and predominantly male world of power. Abraham's paper, it will be remembered, is unclear about whether optimism and generosity arose out of unambivalence in the mother–infant interaction, or out of "excessive indulgence." The first formulation speaks to the positive function of optimism–generosity; the second to its negative functional value. Succorant, nurturant, affiliative (oral) behavior, moreover, is much encouraged in women, in keeping with their role as mothers. Yet these qualities, viewed from the requirements of male competitiveness and aggressiveness, are devalued as "excessive dependency" and passivity. The "oral character" clearly has a different meaning in the life of men and women. Thus, for example, Kagan and Moss (1962) in their longitudinal study have evidence that "passivity and a dependent orientation to adults during childhood showed a remarkable degree of developmental consistency among girls" (p. 72). Girls who were dependent on a female adult at 6 to 10 years old were passive and dependent on a male in adulthood. In contrast to dependency in girls, Kagan and Moss found that the "developmental consistency for aggression was noticeably greater for males" (p. 95). It should be noted, moreover, that Kagan and Moss use the term "dependency" to refer both to "affectional dependency" (positive affiliative behavior) and to "fearful dependency." One finding from their study is of particular interest: Fear of failure in adult females correlated significantly (+.43) with "affectional dependency" (positive orality) in childhood. Women who were closer to their mothers in childhood were more prone to shame of failure in adulthood. In this sense, women's early "orality" apparently predisposed them to increased shame of failure. In any case, as might be predicted from the line of reasoning that suggests different roles for orality in the two sexes, confusing and contradictory sex differences are frequently found in the literature reviews on the oral character.

A second, narrower conceptual difficulty also inheres in Abraham's failure to distinguish between the larger category of emotional ambivalence (or maternal warmth) and quantitative variations along a scale of indulgence–severity. Maternal warmth—or, in its later version, quality of mother–infant interaction—although more difficult to specify quantitatively is likely to be a more powerful predictor of orality than is a single dimension of it, indulgence–severity. As we saw in the case of the anal character, toilet-training procedures were less powerful predictors of adult anal character than mothers' personalities. Similarly, an 18-year longitudinal study of breast- and bottle feeding (Heinstein, 1963) yielded no differences between bottle feeding and breastfeeding in predicting later personality. (Heinstein did find, however, that maternal "warmth" was predictive of good adjustment in both boys and girls.) Other studies of the effect of length of nursing, severity of weaning, and bottle versus cup feeding have yielded negative results. Studies of maternal warmth, and of the quality of the mother–infant interaction, have been more promising predictors (see, e.g., Moss, 1974).

There is, in addition, a methodological difficulty in obtaining data on weaning procedures, namely, the tendency toward retrospective falsification, especially over many years. This point is neatly illustrated in a widely cited early attempt to link adult oral optimism and pessimism to weaning procedures (Goldman-Eisler, 1948, 1950, 1951). Goldman-Eisler first carefully prepared a measure of optimism and pessimism, based on the psychoanalytic literature. In a factor analysis of this instrument, she identified a factor of oral pessimism—and suggested that the psychoanalytic description of this trait be amended to distinguish between "placid" pessimists, who would be unlikely to seek treatment, and "impulsive and aggressive" pessimists, who would be more likely to seek treatment. It is interesting that an "oral pessimist" factor did not show, in keeping with the generally clearer descriptions of "negative"oral states than of "positive" ones.

Having obtained evidence for the existence of oral pessimism among adults, Goldman-Eisler took the next step of inquiring into their early experiences. For this question she asked respondents to inquire of their mothers, and used such retrospective data as the basis for finding a measure of early or late weaning. As she predicted, the information thus indirectly obtained from the mothers correlated with the oral pessimism score. It must be emphasized, however, not only that retrospective data are unreliable, but that there may have been additional aspects of infant feeding, such as sucking on bottles of juice, that Goldman-Eisler's questions to the mothers ignored. Nevertheless, even if retrospective falsification is at work, it is amusing to realize that subjects' accounts of their mothers' weaning procedures still connect (an account of) early weaning with the subjects' own pessimism score. It is not too difficult to imagine that a "pessimism" factor made pessimistic subjects' accounts of their sad weaning fit their generally pessimistic attitudes.

Lines of Development from the Freudian Concept of Orality

Attention to the oral stage of infancy inevitably drew observers to other aspects of the earliest period of life, and from a focus on feeding practices—which did not turn out to be strongly predictive—to broader questions of the affective quality of the mother–infant interaction. Pioneering empirical investigations by Spitz (1945) yielded dramatic evidence that infants separated from their mothers showed evidence not only of acute emotional distress but of severe detriment to the infant's general development. Spitz and Wolf used the term "anaclitic depression" to describe the behavior of these separated infants. "Anaclitic" had been used by Freud to describe a state of "leaning on" or depending upon caretakers for nutritional and other "supplies." Applied to depression, the adjective "anaclitic" retained a strong connection between Spitz's formulation of his results and the Freudian concept of orality.

In later studies, Spitz and Wolf (1946, 1949) observed that infants who were being reared by emotionally ambivalent mothers, from whom they received contradictory positive and negative messages, were likely to display a "rocking" motion as their form of autoerotic behavior, whereas infants who had had relatively unambivalent experiences with their mothers, and were then abruptly separated from them, showed evidence of fecal play as their characteristic erotic behavior. A control group of infants reared under good affectional conditions were more likely to show "genital play" as their autoerotic activity. Spitz and Wolf's finding of fecal play in infants who had presumably formed a good attachment that was then lost was entirely unexpected. They interpreted it as indicating the existence of a loved-hated "introject," who was symbolized by the feces. This finding that infants subject to differences in the affective quality of their relationship to their mothers will find different autoerotic outlets is most important. It suggests that the quality of social-affective interaction in infancy directs the course of autoerotic behavior rather than the reverse, which Freud first suggested. It is not the sexual instinct and its opposition that determines the course of affectional development; rather affectional ties govern the sexual manifestations. This was also a major finding of the Harlows: that maternal deprivation in infancy results in adult sexual incompetence.

During the 1950s Bowlby, following a line of research that began with studies of wartime separation, evolved his concept of a biologically given, goal-corrected attachment system. In this formulation he broke with the concept of orality, and with Freud's drive-reduction theoretical system. Bowlby's systematic studies of maternal deprivation, and the controversy they engendered over "mother love," are still active stimulants to research (see Rutter, 1972, for an excellent review).

Harlow's work on the mother–infant interaction, undertaken in response to the controversies raised by Freudian concepts, opened up another major line of investigation, in which the conditions surrounding rhesus monkey life could be systematically varied in a way not possible with human beings. Severe distress, closely paralleling human infant distress, could be observed in rhesus monkey infants separated from their mothers (Seay, Hansen, & Harlow, 1962). These results were "in general accord with expectations based upon the human separation syndrome described by Bowlby" (p. 132). In their series of studies, the Harlows were able to vary conditions by the introduction of a surrogate mother and by raising monkeys in partial and total isolation, comparing response to peers with response to adults. A recent volume by Harlow and Mears (1979) summarizes the many investigations that have been carried out by Harlow and his team.

Harlow's work has convinced him that

> the so-called primary drives of hunger, fear, rage and pain are actually socially disruptive, and not the proper prerogative on which to form the foundation of behavior of social animals such as men and monkeys. The most fundamental social motives are various forms of love or affection with many comparable components even though men's motives may be more subtle and more persistent. (Harlow & Mears, 1979, p. 8)

The editors of a recent handbook on infancy (Stone, Smith, & Murphy, 1978) summarize these developments in essential agreement with the Harlows. They agree also with Bowlby that

> attachment must be accounted for in its own right. Attempts to derive it [in Freudian theory or in "dependency" theories] from so-called primary drives have fallen of their own weight. . . . It is now widely agreed that babies do not love their mothers because their mothers feed them. (p. 7)

It should be noted, however, that a formulation in terms of "instincts" or drive reduction has been the heritage of Freud's metapsychology, not of his observations. It was Freud's description of the "vicissitudes" of the mother–infant interaction that sparked the investigations that have since overturned his narrower theoretical views.

Whether the theoretical orientation is psychodynamic or behavioral, an uneasy and often unacknowledged consensus exists in modern academic psychology on the proposition that the mother–infant relationship is a powerful and pervasive determinant of personality and cognitive style throughout the course of development. (See Stone *et al.*, 1978, for an excellent summary of an enormous literature.) A listing of some of the robust concepts that have emerged out of the study of infancy will serve to illustrate the great advances that have occurred in our knowledge. Each of these concepts either could have been predicted from psychoanalytic observations, or can readily be assimilated to the social nature of human nature that psychoanalytic observations helped to clarify:

(1) The concept of a "secure base" from which the infant develops self-confidence and exploratory behavior.

(2) The related concepts of "stranger-anxiety," "separation distress," and "joy at reunion" as normal infant responses.

(3) The concept of intrinsically social stimuli, such as the undistorted human face, being picked up when crying, the gentle human voice, and the phenomenal ability of neonates to discriminate speech sounds.

(4) The "social smile," the "smile of effectance" or mastery, as social responses (genetically based) in infancy.

(5) The parallel between the development of perceptual (inanimate) "object constancy" and (person) object constancy, with the question still open which comes first.

(6) "Appropriate caretaking," *creating* "contingencies" out of caretakers' ability to discriminate the difference between infant crying as social protest or physical distress.

(7) The pervasive and powerful sex differences in infant–mother interaction that have been discovered in all these lines of investigation.

One major difference between the present and Freud's time is the development of sophisticated observational methods and the use of advanced technological and statistical tools. Electronic monitoring of neonates' EEGs, videotaping of behavior with the built-in possibility of slow-motion study, techniques for reliable scales, as well as multivariate statistical analysis, now computer assisted, have all developed since the

1940s when Freudian concepts were first being absorbed by academia. The deficiencies of Freud's metapsychology, together with the methodological naïveté of early empirical approaches, combined to create many false starts. Nevertheless, Freud's observations on the dynamics of infancy are being replicated today, and extended to include aspects of infant social capacity that were implied in Kleinian interpretations of his doctrine.

The social capacities of infants are now visible even at birth. For example, infants who are only thirty-six hours old can discriminate and imitate adult facial expressions reflecting happiness, sadness and surprise (Field, Woodson, Greenberg, Cohen, 1982). Newborns can discriminate and prefer the sound of their mothers' voices (DeCasper and Fifer, 1980). These are findings that could not be anticipated by Freud, and they are contrary to his theory of the infant's disorganized and chaotic id. But they are findings that can be assimilated to Freud's observations of the importance of the infant–mother interaction.

One example of a sophisticated statistical study of the mother–infant dyad will illustrate the language in which psychodynamic concepts are now couched (Stern, Caldwell, Hersher, Lipton, & Richmond, 1969). Building on the already recognized parent variables of love–hostility, autonomy–control, and anxious involvement versus calm detachment, Stern *et al.* undertook a factor analytic study of the reciprocal influences of maternal and infant responses. Reliable ratings (a consensus of four observers) were obtained on 30 young mothers and their infants, observed separately and in interaction. Mothers interviewed (with observers using a one-way mirror) during the first trimester of their pregnancy, then again when the baby was 1 year old. For the assessments, scales were evolved that relied on Murray's "needs–press schema," itself a direct inheritor of psychodynamic observations. Among the scales were such polarities as abasement–self-confidence, disorder–orderliness, object versus person orientation, and emotionality–placidity. Among the scales for mothers' handling of their babies were affective involvement, empathy with baby, fastidiousness, cuddling, skill in handling, and enjoyment of baby. Nine infant scales of behavior were also employed, together with a scale of infant intellectual development. From the matrix of intercorrelations among this enormous number of variables, nine common factors were derived. These were found to be intercorrelated in patterns that make excellent psychodynamic sense. For example, one factor "comes close to representing an operational definition of the ideal mother–infant dyad. . . . These are loving, attentive, skillful and involved mothers who impressed the raters by the quality of their mothering" (p. 175). It is interesting that their babies showed accelerated development, a finding reminiscent of Spitz's early observations. On the other side was a factor characterized by a mother's "smug, capricious indifference"; the infant's behavior is similarly "capricious." Still another factor represents mothers whose self-esteem is particularly disturbed and children who have become hostile and disturbed themselves. "The total picture is of mothers whose negative perception of themselves is reinforced by their infants' hostile demandingness" (p. 179).

Not all sophisticated infancy studies, of course, start with Freudian concepts. Some start with a behaviorist learning approach to the mother–infant interaction, as, for example, Watson's (1973) study of the origin of cooing and smiling. Watson describes how two lines of behaviorist research, one into the development of perceptual object orientation and the other into early instrumental learning, led him to an "ethologicosociocognitive hypothesis" which he calls "The Game." (Critics of psychoanalysis for its use of jargon should not neglect the behaviorists' "instrumentalities," "reinforcements," and "contingencies.") Watson suggests that smiling and cooing occur when the infant learns by "contingency analysis" that it can make something happen—for example, it can make a mobile dangling above its crib move by kicking with its feet. Watson cites Hunt and Uzgiris who dubbed the infant's reaction a "smile of effectance." Watson suggests that through this early instrumental competence developed by the infant, adults get involved in the infant's contingency analysis because they begin "playing a game with the infant." They touch his nose each time he widens his eyes, or bounce him on their knee each time he bobs his head, or blow on his belly each time he jiggles his legs, or make sounds after he makes sounds. These games are variants of "The Game." As the infant experiences "clear contingencies"—that he can make people play the game—"vigorous smiling and cooing begin" (p. 108). By the same token, if the situation does not contain clear contingencies, if it is sometimes contingent sometimes not, then "negative emotional responses may occur" (p. 108).

It is significant that "The Game" denotes playfulness. This is a label not only for presumably random adult interventions (such as blowing on the belly every time the infant jiggles his legs), but, as Freud taught us, for affectionate interventions, which are, at the very least, positively toned. Watson's hypothesis explicitly relies heavily not only on contingency analysis (learning) but on built-in genetic propensities. These include that the infant is "specially sensitive and responsive to fellow-members of our species," with built-in schemata for the face and voice. These schemata operate in coordination with the infant's "expectable environment," which necessarily includes the presence of a fellow member of the species. The reference here clearly evokes Hartmann's "average expectable environment."

Watson contrasts his hypothesis with competing ones, such as Bowlby's and Ainsworth's. He neatly pinpoints his central point of difference: " 'The Game' is not important because people play it" but rather "People become important to the infant because they play 'The Game' " (p. 115). In this contrast we see a modern version of the problem Freud faced in his metapsychology. The question was then, as it was for Watson, how the infant becomes hooked up with its caretaker. Freud attached them via the connection that forms (by "contingency analysis") *between the hunger instinct,* that is, the necessity of eating, and the sexual instinct. Watson attaches infant to mother by connecting pleasure in mastery of the physical environment with the pleasure in mastery over the people who are in the environment (and playful). Freud's metapsychology and modern-day behaviorism are agreed in theorizing that the infant is, first of all, an individualist, and social relations evolve out of primary survival mechanisms such as eating or instrumental learning. Other students of infancy, in contrast, conceptualize social relations as the infant's primary survival mechanism. But even in the behaviorist stronghold a concept of some "given" social sensitivity to people is acknowledged as required by the evidence.

FREUD'S LIBIDINAL TYPES, SEX DIFFERENCES, AND FIELD-DEPENDENT COGNITIVE STYLE

In a very short paper, written relatively late, after his struggles with his structural theory, Freud (1931) tentatively suggested three psychological types that could comprehend not only the familiar clinical populations but normal people as well. Fifteen years earlier, in a better-known paper on characterological types encountered in analytic work, Freud (1916) described people whose character is determined essentially by their sense of guilt (or innocence). Some people refuse to tolerate the privations of analysis because they are "exceptions"—they have already been unjustly treated. Others are wrecked by success, because of their "sense of guilt"; still others commit criminal acts out of a "sense of guilt." Freud's attention had clearly been turned by 1916 to a closer examination of the "forces of shame, disgust and morality" which oppose the sexual instinct.

In his 1931 paper he based his typology, interestingly enough, not directly on his metapsychology but on the "libidinal situation," even though, as discussed in Volume 1, he had reluctantly abandoned the libido theory of anxiety in 1926. Once again his ambivalence about libido theory is apparent. The three types in the 1931 paper are put forward almost apologetically: "[They] will hardly escape the suspicion of having been deduced from the theory of the libido" (p. 218).

Although Freud also found it difficult to name his types, he settled on calling them the *erotic*, the *narcissistic*, and the *obsessional*. Each of these is a "pure type"; the central point of each type is the extent to which the libido is "predominantly allocated to the provinces of the mental apparatus" (p. 217). (The provinces are the id, ego, and super-ego.) What is at issue in each type is the way in which the self relates to other people, either directly—the erotic type—or via the self's relation to its conscience—the obsessional type—or else the self relates to others very little—the narcissistic type. The text of Freud's descriptions follows.

> The *erotic* type is easily characterized. Erotics are those whose main interest—the relatively largest part of whose libido—is turned towards love. Loving, but above all, being loved is the important thing for them. They are dominated by the fear of loss of love and are therefore especially dependent on others who may withhold their love from them. . . . From the social and cultural standpoint this type represents the elementary instinctual demands of the id, to which the other psychical agencies have become compliant.
>
> The second type is what I have termed the *obsessional* type—a name which may at first seem strange. It is distinguished by the predominance of the superego which is separated from the ego under great tension. People of this type are dominated by fear of their conscience instead of fear of losing love. They exhibit, as it were, an internal instead of an external dependence. They develop a high degree of self-reliance; and, from the social standpoint, they are the true, preeminently conservative vehicles of civilization.
>
> The third type, justly called the *narcissistic*, is mainly to be described in negative terms. There is no tension between the ego and the superego (indeed, on the strength of this type one would scarcely have arrived at the hypothesis of a superego), and there is no preponderance of erotic needs. The subject's main interest is directed to self-preservation; he is independent and not open to intimidation. His ego has a large amount of aggressiveness at his disposal, which also manifests itself in readiness for activity. In his erotic life loving is preferred over being loved. People who belong to this type impress others as being "personalities"; they are especially suited to act as a support for others, to take on the role of leaders and to give a fresh stimulus to cultural development or to damage the established state of affairs. (p. 218)

After describing these three pure types, Freud proceeds to a discussion of mixtures of the three, frequently observed in analysis. Then, as if it were a "jest" (derived from his own obsessionality), Freud asks: Why not postulate a mixed style of erotic-narcissistic-obsessional people? He quickly moves away from his own "jest" to give a serious answer: these people would be "the absolute norm, the ideal harmony" (p. 219), obviously representing the union of id, ego, and superego. Such a formulation of an "ideal" does not take us much beyond the obvious.

It is also clear that Freud's description of his three types implies a sex difference, with women falling in the erotic-narcissistic type and men falling in the erotic-obsessional type. As we saw in the chapter on sex differences, Freud was convinced of the narcissistic nature of women. He speculates, for example, that people of the erotic-narcissistic type have a tendency to hysteria if they fall ill, whereas obsessionals are more prone to obsessional neurosis, a reference to the clearly observed sex differences in proneness to these illnesses.

In any case, a typology based on the mode of relatedness between the self and others has a sweep that goes beyond the details of early feeding and toileting. The emphasis is on the relationship between the self and significant others, whether in the threat of "loss of love" or in "fear of conscience." The resulting characterology involves dependency on others in the former and "internal rather than external dependency" in the latter.

The similarity between this line of character description and the cognitive style of field dependence is self-evident. But the historical connection with the development of Witkin's concepts and Freudian thinking is indirect rather than direct. As we saw in Chapter 6, New Look investigators during the 1950s were busy attempting to evolve experimental situations in which Freudian defenses and developmental phases could be put to test. In this atmosphere, Witkin's "accidental" discovery of what turned out to be stable and significant differences in people's perception of the upright in space could be used to test Freudian thinking. A person whose mode of orienting in space was "self-centered" could be expected to have a personality that fit this cognitive style. Here was, in other words, a ready-made opportunity, which Witkin grasped, to use a robust perceptual performance as a "tracer element" in the study of the self in its manifold relation to others and to the world.

The perceptual problem on which Witkin was working at the time of his discovery was a specific formulation of a larger problem raised by the Gestalt psychologist Max Wertheimer as early as 1912. Wertheimer puzzled over the question whether the self should be understood as an "egotistical" product or as a product of interaction with the "field." Gestalt theory, with its emphasis on the organization of the field rather than on random stimulus–response connections, would predict that even the perception of the upright in space was not an egotistical product but a function of the self in relation to the organization of the field.

Wertheimer had observed that two sets of experimental factors ordinarily come together to make it possible for us to determine with great accuracy how far our bodies are "off" from the true vertical, and how far objects are off from their usual framework. Under ordinary circumstances kinesthetic feedback from the pull of gravity on the body combines with visual perception of the verticals and horizontals in space to give us a large fund of information on which we base our automatic and very accurate judgments of the position of the body and of objects in space. Wertheimer designed a method of separating the visual from the postural cues in the perception of the upright, predicting that a test of their relative potency would favor the visual framework over the ("self-centered") body cues as the more potent determinant. Wertheimer's original experiment had confirmed his hypothesis; later experiments by Gibson and Mowrer (1938) had contradicted Wertheimer's findings. Asch and Witkin (1948) and Witkin and Asch (1948) were attempting to reconcile this discrepancy when Witkin made his observations about individual differences (the most probable reason for the discrepancy). It should be noted that, in the main, Wertheimer's hypothesis has been confirmed: People do tend on the average to be influenced by the prevailing visual framework in their perception of the upright in space.

The fact that there are individual differences in the perception of the body's position in space was quite unpredicted by Gestalt theory, which emphasized the compelling nature of a visual framework of organization for everyone. But it did fit a psychodynamic way of thinking in which the self's relation to others, and to the world, is the inheritor of oral and anal developmental phases as well as of "tensions between ego and superego."

The team of investigators Witkin assembled to study individual differences in the perception of the upright included psychoanalytically trained psychologists, of whom I was one (Witkin, Lewis, Hertzman, Machover, Meissner, & Wapner, 1954). During the pilot phase of our study, I undertook to guess from a clinical interview who would line up a stick with the tilted frame and who would align it with the true vertical whatever the tilt of the surrounding framework. Choosing out of a great welter of impressions was indeed difficult, but successful blind guesses could be made on the basis of whether the person impressed us as having a strong, not to say disagreeable, self, or a more accommodating and compliant self. The early discovery of a small but statistically significant difference between the sexes in the direction expected from stereotypical sex roles was another congruence with Freudian theory. The first team of investigators was able to establish significant correlations among the Rod and Frame Test, the Body Adjustment Test, and the Rotating Room Test of perception of the upright, as well as the Embedded Figures Test, which taps "disembedding," but not in the context of perceiving the upright in space. Correlations were predicted and confirmed between these perceptual tests and scores derived from a clinical interview, the Rorschach, the TAT, and drawings of the human figure. In short, the way the self responded to the framework was congruent with the person's style of responding to others, as measured by a psychoanalytically based interview and projective tests.

A developmental study of field dependence in 10-year-old boys (Witkin, Dyk, Goodenough, Faterson, & Karp, 1962) extended the range of analytical abilities related to field dependence and established a connection between mother's emphasis on personal autonomy and her son's field dependence. A mother of a field-dependent boy was more likely to have attitudes that encouraged her son's continued association with her, as expressed by her limiting the child's activities in the community, emphasizing conformity, discouraging aggressive and assertive behavior (particularly when directed against herself), and not stimulating the child to assume responsibilities. Parents of field-dependent boys also used more severe methods of discipline in controlling them. These findings are confirmed in cross-cultural studies showing clearly that obedience and conformity are associated with field dependency (Berry, 1976).

The continuity of an individual's field-dependent cognitive style has been established experimentally, from age 10 to adulthood. The network of correlations that can be put together meaningfully from field dependence as a center touches literally all areas of psychology, from cerebral hemisphere specialization, to shame and guilt, to obedience in agrarian versus hunter–gatherer economies. Field dependence has turned out to be such a powerful tool because it has established a relationship between the self's response to the inanimate or physical world and its response to emotionally significant others. I have suggested (Lewis, 1976) that these are the two main tracks of the self's relation to the nonself. These two areas of the nonself make very different demands upon the organization of the self. In emotional relationships, the boundaries between the self and the other are necessarily fluid; what affects the other person also affects the self in empathic and vicarious experiences. In response to the physical world, the self's boundaries in relation to the nonself must be sharper and more articulated.

That stable emotional attachments formed early should predict a self that is interpersonally adept *and* field independent is, of course, a central tenet of psychoanalytic thinking. The stability of emotional attachments is expected to predict "good" things both affectively and cognitively. But the evidence from the work on field dependence does not bear out this agreeable assumption. Even in early childhood, and especially among boys, there is evidence that field independence goes together with an orientation toward objects rather than people. (For a careful review of this question see Kogan, 1976.) There is, in fact, strong evidence for the paradox that field independence goes with cognitive restructuring skills but with deficits in dealing interpersonally, whereas field dependence goes with interpersonal skills but with cognitive restructuring deficits.

It is when we look at the evidence on sex differences in field dependence in early childhood, and put it together with the evidence on what affective factors are connected with intellectual development, that we begin to shed some light on the paradox. Even in preschool children, there is a sex difference in field dependence. (The Preschool Embedded Figures Test or the Children's Embedded Figures Test are among the measures employed.) But the sex difference before age 5 goes mainly in the opposite direction: Little girls are more field independent than little boys, especially at age 5. When this finding is brought together with the evidence about the sex differences in personality factors that are associated with intellectual development in children, we see that an optimal level of intellectual functioning is associated with girls being assertive and active and having a sense that they can "control their own actions," whereas for boys, who are "already sufficiently assertive," the important issue in intellectual development is how well they control their aggressive impulses" (Maccoby & Jacklin, 1974, p. 133). This package of evidence, moreover, fits the general finding that, for men, being treated with maternal warmth in childhood, and becoming "cautious," well-controlled children, makes for higher IQ in adulthood. For women, in contrast, the crucial experience fostering intellectual development is having a mother who allows them relative freedom from restrictions; "impulsive" little girls, for example, are better at tasks involving analytical ability. In any case, it can be supposed that little girls are closer to the "optimal conditions" during their preschool years because of their lesser aggressivity in general (Maccoby & Jacklin, 1974) and the greater ease with which their early socialization progresses (Sears, Rau, & Alpert, 1965; Moss, 1974).

By the time children reach school age, however, the differing demands that the socialization makes on them—for boys the requirement that they cultivate more cognitive skills, for girls that they cultivate their interpersonal skills—result in reversing the relationship between the two sexes. Thus, in a way reminiscent of the way Freud's findings on hysteria in women led to a critique of society, the work on field dependence helps to clarify the way our social order demands different sacrifices from the two sexes.

That cognition is distorted by unbearable affect is a Freudian discovery that still dominates the modern psychology of personality, although the when and how of affective power over cognition is still mysterious. Freud's influence has been enormous in the field of personality assessment, in ways that would require volumes to document. Freudian influence, however, has varied in its direction with the divisions within the psychoanalytic movement. In particular, Hartmann's "ego psychology" has tended to mute Freud's description of the affective basis for behavior, whereas the "object-relations" approach continues to emphasize it.

FREUDIAN INFLUENCE ON PERSONALITY ASSESSMENT

As we saw in Chapter 5, Hartmann's emendation of Freud's metapsychology—the "conflict-free ego-sphere"—simply concedes that affect is not always all-powerful, a stipulation that Freud always emphasized in his descriptive accounts. But the fact remains that affects are very powerful even in such strongholds of "ego" function as locomotion or handwriting. Walking, for example, is a maturational function whose rate of development is relatively uninfluenced by the parent–child affective interaction (putting aside, for the moment, observations by Ainsworth, 1963, about the early age of locomotion among closely bonded Uganda infants). But the differences in the characteristic gait of individuals are very striking. One recognizes intimates easily by the characteristic sound of their walk. What is more, gait and carriage tell us much about such major characteristics of personal style as vigor and gender. The majority of us in developed countries learn to write, following a set of cognitive prescriptions for rendering language into script. But handwritings are so uniquely characteristic that graphologists can discern personal styles and identify individuals from their writing. Reading personality from gait or script clearly reflects that these "routinely" learned functions carry the precipitates of personal affective struggles in the form of a cognitive style.

As we see in these two examples, the concept of a cognitive style implies an organized self, functioning to maintain its affective relations to others, so that even routine performances bear an affective-personal cognitive imprint. This is an essentially Freudian concept although it found unclear expression in Freud because of his failure to conceptualize the self as a social process. Its clear expression is also muted in Hartmann's concept of an "autonomous" ego.

The concept of an affectively based cognitive style in which the self functions defensively to maintain its affectional ties is basic to all the varieties of "projective" methods of assessing personality. In this sense, Freud's ideas have been incorporated into the major forms of psychological assessment in current use. In contrast to projective tests, which are rooted in psychoanalytic theory, there are, of course, the theoretically neutral empirical instruments, such as the MMPI and Eysenck's Neuroticism Scale. These are essentially self-reports of symptoms complexes, such as anxiety, worry, hypochondria, or depression. Their content does not differ descriptively from the phenomena with which Freud was dealing. The demonstrated usefulness of these instruments, which is sometimes interpreted as evidence against psychoanalytic thinking, actually speaks to the correctness of Freud's clinical observations about symptoms.

It is fascinating to observe how the history of projective testing itself follows the development of thinking within the psychoanalytic movement, from the first "word-association" test, Jung's measure of the invaded "ego," through Rorschach's reliance on primitive imagery, and back again to modern hierarchical measures of ego development (e.g., Loevinger, 1976). Beginning with Jung's Free Association Test, which constructed an assessment procedure out of the ideational-associative web reflecting unconscious conflict, projective tests have relied on Freud's unraveling of the content of symptoms and dreams. But they have varied in how directly or indirectly "secondary process" is involved. Rorschach's (1921/1946) test, which followed on Jung's, studied the affective character of cognition by requiring responses to visual images that were themselves either ambiguous or meaningless unless organized into affective-cognitive symbols. The visual images in Rorschach's inkblots were meant to represent the unconscious also in being nonverbal stimuli. Note that the "unconscious" in Rorschach's formulation is either ambiguous or meaningless, a conception that tends to denigrate the cognitive sense of affects. Rorschach's purpose was to

> follow the conflict between the repressing conscious and the repressed unconscious, and observe how the neurotic repression narrows the productive sphere and see how the freedom of "inner life" is completely stifled by conscious restraints (corrections) and by compulsive super-criticisms. (p. 203)

Murray's Thematic Apperception Test, as developed by Tomkins, allowed much more of cognitive content into the assessment stimulus, although the pictorial scenes were also designed for the ambiguousness of their affective content. The analysis of responses to the pictorial scenes involved an assessment of personality according to how needs were handled, the needs being essentially versions of Freudian psychosexual stages: *n* succorance, *n* nurturance, *n* achievement, and the like. Ambiguous pictures were assessed also for oedipal content (Blum, 1963) and for intropunitive versus extrapunitive defenses (Rosenzweig, 1938). This latter focus has been very fruitful.

Following Hartmann's formulation of a conflict-free ego-sphere, Rorschach's interpretation was revised to prevent it from becoming "wild," and to bring Rorschach research in line with the developments of ego-psychology (Schafer, 1954). In particular, the nature of the relationship between the tester and the client as reflected in Rorschach responses was reassessed. Rorschach responses were reevaluated not only for their place on a continuum from "primitive" dream content to the "objective, realistic percept-like responses at the progressive secondary process role" (p. 90), but the responses could "simultaneously bear the imprint of primitive, unrealistic, unconscious processes and articulated, realistic, conscious processes" (p. 92).

By the early sixties Gottschalk and Gleser (1969) had evolved a method of assessing implied effective content from "ordinary" verbal samples. A clause-by-clause analysis of verbal content, using Freudian assumptions, identifies six variables of anxiety—death, separation, mutilation, shame, guilt, and diffuse anxiety—and three modes of hostility—outward, inward, and ambivalently directed. This method of analysis of verbal content is highly reliable and has proved to be a valid discriminator of the presence and intensity of anxiety and hostility. In keeping with "ego-psychological" concepts, Gleser and Ihilevich (1969) and Loevinger (1976) have developed assessment scales that make direct use of people's ordinary ideation about life situations, but still assess the covert ways in which people defend themselves against unbearable affects. The pendulum has thus swung back and forth between the id and the ego as assessment techniques traveled from word associations, through Rorschachs and TATs, and back again to Hartmann-influenced verbal measures of ego development. The problem of relating cognition to affect in a cognitive style or an affective style clearly remains central.

CHAPTER 8

Totem and Taboo
The Problem of the Origins of Guilt and Civilization

Freud's interest in the origins of guilt came relatively late in his work, as he himself acknowledged (1933). It was only after his major clinical accounts had been written that Freud undertook a study of the origins of guilt in *Totem and Taboo*. In his clinical papers, as well as in his books on dreams and jokes, "disgust, shame, and morality" were simply the counterforces against which sexual longings (libido) contended. Moreover, the origin of these counterforces was at first located in the sexual instincts themselves (see Chapter 4) as sublimations and reaction formations of the sexual instincts. Hostility arose out of frustrated libido; sublimations and reaction formations of hostility (although in the service of the "ego-instincts") also made use of the energy of the sexual instincts to deflect them into social and moral purposes. In this account, libido theory is the centerpiece of the explanation. Our path might have been easier if Freud had indeed regarded his libido theory as a theory of the emotions (as he said he did in *Group Psychology*, 1921, p. 90). If one permits libido to stand for the attachment emotions, the origin of hostility and morality in a single source becomes a viable hypothesis. Morality is the affective-cognitive outcome of attachment. Threatened attachment, which first evokes protest aimed at the caretaker—"other," is then transformed, mainly by identification, into states of shame and guilt that aim at maintaining the attachment.

Reading *Totem and Taboo* 70 years after it was written, one is struck by the irony that one of its most important, seminal ideas—the idea that identification is the source of guilt—was almost buried in what now seem like trivial controversies over the historical reality of the primal deed, or the existence of a collective unconscious. These controversies reflect the epistemological uncertainty (still existing today) of anchoring emotions in "reality." Freud did not highlight the concept of identification, which had and still has little theoretical clarity. Yet its power to predict many phenomena in cross-cultural studies of human socialization is one outcome that this chapter and the next will document. In cross-cultural studies undertaken by psychoanalytically oriented anthropologists, as well as in the work of such Freudian critics as Lévi-Strauss and Piaget, identification of one human being with another has been a central psychological assumption.

Freud's psychoanalytic treatises on the origins of guilt, religion (1927a) and civilization (1930) were all written in a materialist philosophical tradition. For example, in order to convey the special insights that psychoanalysis can bring to bear upon the explanation of taboos, Freud contrasted his materialist views with those of a leading psychologist of his time—none other than Wilhelm Wundt. Freud quotes Wundt's version of the sources of taboo: " 'They have their origin in the source of the most primitive and at the same time the most lasting of human instincts—in fear of "demonic" powers' " (1913, p. 24). He expresses disappointment in Wundt's explanation:

> Neither fear nor demons can be regarded by psychology as "earliest" things, impervious to any attempt at discovering their antecedents. It would be another thing if demons *really existed*. But we know that, like gods, they are creations of the human mind; they were made by something out of something. (p. 24, italics added)

As we can see in this passage, Freud's criticism of Wundt would be welcomed by any critic of instinct theory. Clearly Freud is looking to experiential factors for his explanations; even more important, he is determined to base taboo within materialist philosophy—upon things that exist rather than on an instinctive fear of nonexistent demonic powers.

A main theme of *Totem and Taboo* is the idea of the unity of the human psyche, specifically the universality of guilt. The subtitle for *Totem and Taboo* is *Some Points of Agreement between the Mental Life of Savages and Neurotics:*

> It may begin to dawn on us that the taboos of the average Polynesians are after all not so remote from us as we were inclined to think at first, that the moral and conventional prohibitions by which we ourselves are governed

may have some essential relationship with these primitive taboos and that an explanation of taboo might throw some light on the obscure origin of our own "categorical imperative". (1913, p. 22)

Freud was consciously a pioneer in his interdisciplinary approach to the problem of guilt. He was especially drawn to anthropology by the phenomenological similarity between accounts of primitive taboos and "Kant's 'categorical imperative', which [also] operates in a compulsive fashion and rejects any conscious motives" (1913, p. xiv). In his assumption of morality as a universal human psychological structure, Freud actually anticipated the thinking of many modern anthropologists, most notably Lévi-Strauss, an avowed critic of Freud. Lévi-Strauss, without specifically saying so, clearly agrees with Freud that the incest taboo is the hallmark of humanity. He writes:

If social organization had a beginning, this could only have consisted in the incest prohibition . . . since the incest prohibition is, in fact, a kind of remodeling of the biological conditions of mating and procreation. . . . It is there, and only there, that we find a passage from nature to culture, from animal to human life. (1969, p. 278)

As we shall see again in the next chapter, Lévi-Strauss, although vociferously anti-Freudian, shares many of Freud's ideas, as well as his androcentric bias.

Freud, however, contradicted his own assumption of the unity of the human psyche in also assuming that a hierarchy of rationality exists in which neurotics, savages, women, and children are inferior to civilized adult men. The contradiction in his thinking on this point is very clear when we contrast his admiration and surprise at the complexity of primitive incest taboos with his disdain for their infantile affectivity. On the one hand, Freud praises the intellectual powers of savages (a stance that Lévi-Strauss has so fully elaborated). Freud regrets the underestimation of savages' "fullness and delicacy of feeling" (p. 99). He is surprised that

the sexual life of these poor naked cannibals . . . would be moral in our sense or that their sexual instincts would be subjected to any great degree of restriction. Yet we find that they set before themselves with the most scrupulous care and the most painful severity the aim of avoiding incestuous relations. Indeed, their whole social organization seems to serve that purpose or to have been brought into relation with its attainment. (p. 2)

On the other hand, Freud regards the unusually great horror of incest among savages as an "*infantile* feature . . . in striking agreement with the mental life of neurotic patients" (p. 17). By implication, the horror of incest is a remnant of civilization's historical past. People caught in the throes of strong affect, instead of reason, are *ipso facto* less truly civilized.

Freud thus seems to be suggesting that very strong affects, such as horror, are primitive or neurotic. In this line of thinking incest can be considered an outmoded sexual convention. Some present-day social scientists have suggested, in fact, that incest is an outmoded prohibition (Cohen, 1978), and others, writing in the name of Freudian sexual liberation, have suggested that children have a right to sexual experience with their adult caretakers (Haeberle, 1978; Pomeroy, 1976). Freud's position that horror or intense guilt is an expendable (primitive, irrational) state thus involves a contradiction with his idea that guilt (including intense guilt) is a necessity of civilization.

This contradiction remains unsolved to this day. Recently, for example, students of the Holocaust have had to confront the notion that extreme horror is not *ipso facto* neurotic but may be appropriate to the extreme dehumanization of Holocaust conditions. In a study of the children of Holocaust survivors, Wilson and Fromm (in press) discovered that many of them were burdened by survivor guilt, as if they and not their parents had been the direct survivors. Thus a number of these second-generation adults were plagued by "anniversary reactions" to Holocaust events, during which they made "compassionate sacrifices" of their own welfare for the sake of their survivor parents. The (now adult) children were reluctant to enter preferred psychotherapy because of a need to feel protective toward their parents, and especially to emphasize the heroic aspects of their parents' past. They avoided therapy since it might threaten their attachment to their parents. Wilson and Fromm found it difficult to use any of the current psychoanalytic paradigms in trying to understand guilt in second-generation survivors, primarily because survivor guilt tends to be regarded as *ipso facto* neurotic. Second-generation survivor guilt may, however, appropriately bear witness to an extraordinary evil—a total eclipse of attachment emotions—which cannot and should not be forgotten, lest it recur. Similarly, the horror of incest can be regarded as an appropriate reaction to the betrayal of a child's trust that adult power will not be abused, as well as to the betrayal of a child's affection in sexual arousal. A strong horror reaction to the subversive destruction of the attachment emotions is not *ipso facto* neurotic.

In focusing on the "categorical imperative" as his model of morality, Freud was also narrowing the range of moral experience that can be regarded as universal. The "categorical imperative" as the model for morality is particularly congenial to an industrial society requiring the autonomy and independence of its individual (male) members (Tawney, 1926; Weber, 1958). Kant's internal "gendarme" (which Marx said every Prussian carries within himself) reflects a juridical model. But as the

Edels have suggested in *Anthropology and Ethics* (1968), there are many other models of morality, both historically and cross-culturally. As one example, ancient Greek society has been described as a "shame" culture in which the strongest moral force is respect for the opinion of others (Dodds, 1951). In contrast, the Bible has been analyzed as reflecting a guilt culture (Daube, 1969). Benedict (1946) traced the importance of shame in contemporary Japanese culture. As still another example, the Kabyle of North Africa describe their moral code as that of "an individual who sees himself always through the eyes of others and who has need of others for his existence, because the image he has of himself is indistinguishable from that presented to him by other people" (Bourdieu, 1966). The Kabyle have a proverb that says, "Man is man through men; God alone is God through himself." Other moral codes focus on individual self-fulfillment as the criterion of morality; still others focus on the decision-making process within a conflict of values (A. Edel, 1980).

Within the psychoanalytic movement, a controversy over whether the ego-ideal (the good) has equal value with the superego (the ought) has been one result of Freud's narrow focus on the categorical imperative (Lewis, 1971; Lynd, 1958; Piers & Singer, 1953; Turiel, 1967). Still another resultant has been the controversy over Freud's view of women's superego as "less impersonal" and therefore less highly developed than men's (Gilligan, 1981; Haan, 1978; Lewis, 1976).

Freud sought the origins of morality not in God-given laws but in the Darwinian concept of adaptation to the conditions of existence. In particular, Freud based his thinking on Darwin's hypothesis that primal society was organized around a dominant male who excluded male juveniles from the troop, thus fostering exogamous matings. Freud's reliance on Darwin is worth illustrating at some length. "Darwin," wrote Freud, "deduced from the habits of the higher apes that men, too, originally lived in comparatively small groups or hordes, within which the jealousy of the oldest and strongest male prevented sexual promiscuity." Freud then quotes Darwin's own words (Darwin, 1871, p. 362f.):

> We may conclude from what we know of the jealousy of all male quadrupeds, armed as many of them are, with special weapons for battling with their rivals, that promiscuous intercourse in a state of nature is extremely improbable. . . . Therefore, if we look far enough back in the stream of time . . . judging from the social habits of man as he now exists . . . the most probable view is that primeval man aboriginally lived in small communities, each with as many wives as he could support and obtain, whom he jealously guarded against all other men. Or he may have lived with several wives by himself, like the gorilla; for all natives agree "that but one adult male is seen in a band; when the young male grows up, a contest takes place

> for mastery, and the strongest, by licking and driving out the others, establishes himself as the head of the community." [Darwin here quotes Dr. Savage, in the *Boston Journal of Natural History*, 1845–1847, 5, p. 423.] The younger males, being thus expelled, and wandering about, would, when at last successful in finding a partner, prevent too close inbreeding within the limits of the same family. (Freud, 1913, p. 125)

Freud's concept of primordial human society was thus of an agonic, male-dominated horde. A number of constraints inhere in this Darwinian concept, as we saw in earlier chapters. The first of these is the focus on the (male) aggression necessary for species survival. The role of tender or affectionate emotions in the evolution of guilt is much underplayed. "Libido" loses its central role and is replaced by aggression, since it is the aggression between males over the supply of females that must somehow be curbed if civilization is to exist.

We now know, as we saw in previous chapters, that there are many different kinds of social organization among primates, depending in great part on differing ecologies (Martin & Voorhies, 1975). Male dominance is not the only factor determining primate social organization. The behavior and the reactions of females have simply been neglected in accounts of primate society (Bernstein, 1978).

A second constraint on the Darwinian model is that women's role in the formation of morality simply does not arise. Not only are the emotions of women not a significant factor in the evolution of guilt, but tender and affectionate feelings in both sexes are relegated to second place.

As we shall see from a careful reading of *Totem and Taboo*, Freud took his clinical insights into the emotions that are behind both the incest taboo and totem ceremonials, and used them to formulate a historical reconstruction of the origin of guilt. Civilized morality began when the sons' acts of parricide and cannibalism were followed by their remorse, and when the incest taboo appeared. But Freud did not permit himself to rely on the sons' conflict between affection and hatred in his theory of the creation of guilt. In his materialist view, the emotions were somehow insufficiently anchored in "reality" to be credited with their own powers. For example, Freud vacillated painfully over the issue of the "reality" of the primal deed, but concluded (tentatively) that it was safer to use the model of an obsessional's guilt, which always rests on an actual evil deed in childhood (1913). In this choice, however, he was actually contradicting his own clinical observation that obsessionals had *not*, in fact, ever committed acts so dreadful as their strong sense of guilt implied. (See Volume 1, Chapter 4 for a description of the dialogue between Freud and the Rat Man in which Freud concedes precisely this point.) But the advantage of basing emotions, which Freud clearly conceived of as "physical," on some "historical" or "factual" reality was too strong for Freud to resist. So, for example, in one passage at the end of *Totem and Taboo*, he puts forth the view that "the mere existence of a wishful *phantasy* of killing him [the father] would have been enough to produce the moral reaction that created totemism and taboo" (p. 160). He goes on to say that the

> distinction [between psychical and factual reality] does not in our judgment affect the heart of the matter. If wishes and impulses have the full value of fact for primitive men, it is our business to give their attitude our understanding attention instead of correcting it in accordance with our own standards.

Clearly, however, "our own standards" require making a distinction between wishes and facts. It should be noted that the problem Freud confronts is created by his making the terms "fantasy" and "wish" synonymous with "emotions," which are then, by implication, events that somehow did not "really occur" but were only "felt." In this concept, emotions, fantasies, and wishes thus have neither veridical cognitive content nor any real power.

Freud's adherence to materialism brought him into difficulties when it came to explaning the transmission of guilt after the primal deed. In order to explain how each generation maintains the incest taboo, he postulated a hereditary transmission of a (suddenly acquired) characteristic. Since he refused to accept the primal deed as an allegory, reflecting universal human emotions, and preferred to accept Lamarckian transmission, *Totem and Taboo* easily became the target of critics for its unscientific assumptions. Even though Freud later (1930) retracted his insistence on the reality of the primal deed, he accompanied this retraction by anchoring guilt in a conflict between two instincts, eros and death. His description of the origin of guilt in a conflict between affection and hatred was once again entangled in a theoretical obscurity—this one created by a reliance on instincts (whose use by Wundt he had so sharply criticized).

In the absence of a viable theory of emotions as real psychological events, Freud contradicted himself frequently about which psychological forces he called "internal" and which "external." Thus in *Thoughts on War and Death* (1915c) he calls the "human need for love" an "internal" factor. In contrast, the force exerted by "upbringing, which represents the claims of our cultural environment" is an "external factor." Throughout an individual's life, Freud goes on to say, there is a "replacement of external by internal compulsion" (p. 282).

On the very next page, however, Freud contradicts himself as to which are internal forces and which external. "Benefits in the way of

love" become "external forces," included with other factors in upbringing. Similarly, in *Civilization and Its Discontents* (1930), "loss of love" is
regarded as an "external" force:

> Originally, renunciation of instinct was the result of fear of an external au-
> thority: one renounced one's satisfactions in order not to lose its love. . . . A
> threatened *external* unhappiness—loss of love and punishment on the part of
> the external authority—has been exchanged for a permanent *internal* unhap-
> piness, for the tension of the sense of guilt. (pp. 127–128, italics added)

This difficulty in ascribing the locus of forces within or without the
organism is the product of an inadequate theory of emotions. If emotions are conceptualized as social processes occurring in the interaction
between people, they are all neither internal nor external. Their apparent locus as "internal" or "external" depends on the presence or absence of imagery of the significant other involved in the interaction. One
result of Freud's treatment of "loss of love" as an "external" force was a
later extrapolation from his writings that shame, a reaction to "loss of
love," is a lower-order or more primitive experience than guilt. This
hierarchy had negative consequences for psychoanalytic therapy; it also
fostered a one-sided view of the nature of morality itself (A. Edel, 1980;
Gilligan, 1981; Lewis, 1976).

Freud was also hampered by an unclarity as to whether the sense of
guilt should be interpreted cognitively, as he usually did, or whether it
should have its more directly affective meaning. This unclarity is reflected in his interchangeable use of the terms *Schuldbewusstsein*, meaning "sense of guilt," and *Schuldgefühl* meaning "feeling of guilt." The
editors of the *Standard Edition* tell us that the second of the two terms is
what Freud uses for the most part, but that they have translated both as
"sense of guilt" because the terms are "synonymous" (1930, p. 135 fn.).

It is also clear that Freud regards "remorse" as an affective state
originating in affectionate feelings for the father. Remorse is the result of
"the primordial ambivalence of feeling toward the father." Freud is
eloquent on the subject of remorse and its role in the origin of conscience. "Now, I think, we can at least grasp two things perfectly clearly: the part played by love in the origin of conscience and the fatal
inevitability of the sense of guilt" (1930, p. 132). Although he actually
attributes great power to this *feeling* of remorse, as a reflection of the
ambivalence between the eros and death instincts (p. 132), he nevertheless insists that remorse is only an instance of the more general and
more important cognitive "sense of guilt." It is this cognitive sense of
guilt that is the "cause of instinctual renunciation to begin with" (p.
128). Freud thus blunts his own statement of the positive affects in-

volved—that it was "remorse for the deed [that] set up the superego by identification with the father" (p. 132).

Freud is also required to

> defend the paradoxical statement that conscience is the result of instinctual renunciation, or that instinctual renunciation (imposed on us from without) creates conscience, which then demands further instinctual renunciation. (p. 129)

This is the same position to which he was driven in *Inhibitions, Symptoms and Anxiety* (1926), namely, that anxiety is the *cause* of repression, rather than its result. Freud was then speaking of the more cognitive sense of anxiety as a "signal of danger." Similarly, the "sense of guilt" is a signal of the existence of the superego—an institution principally of the mind, rather than of emotions, such as remorse.

In summary, then, Freud's thinking on the origin of guilt was hampered by the absence of a viable theory of differentiated emotions. A theory of emotions as attachment phenomena diminishes the separation between rational or cognitive and affective events. It broadens the model of moral experience beyond Kant's categorical imperative. It specifically adds the hedonic mode of social organization to the agonic mode in considering the origin of morality. In so doing, it broadens to include women's experience in the model of morality. A viable theory of emotions helps also to solidify an epistemological basis for emotions in reality.

Let us now look closely at the text of *Totem and Taboo* to see in detail how these issues emerge.

TOTEM AND TABOO

At the time when Freud wrote *Totem and Taboo,* social philosophers and anthropologists of the day were struggling to understand the significance of the complicated and varying kinship systems symbolized by clans and their totems. In particular, there was a debate over the relationship between "totemism," that is, the often elaborate customs and ceremonials surrounding a clan's totem, and exogamy, the rules dictating marriage outside the clan. Some anthropologists, such as Frazer (whom Freud greatly admired), had come to the conclusion (with which Freud disagreed) that totemism and exogamy were entirely independent of each other and had become historically connected only by chance. Others, like Durkheim, saw exogamy as growing out of totemism, with proscriptions arising against a man mating with someone of his own "blood." Durkheim had, in fact, come to the conclusion that the institutions of totemism symbolically represented the community to which people belonged, with exogamy being an inevitable outgrowth of totemic laws. Exogamy was thus beginning to be understood as an institution for the prevention of incest (Freud, 1913, p. 121).

Into this complicated interrelation among totemism, exogamy, and the incest taboo, Freud offered the insights that psychoanalysis might bring. His hypothesis connected totemism, exogamy, and the incest taboo into a single system of familial-emotional relationships evolving out of the Darwinian horde. The psychoanalytic observations came from obsessional neurosis, the illness in which guilt is rampant, and phobia, in which anxiety is uncontrollable. The universal origins lay in the incest taboo, which constituted a basic difference between ourselves and our primate ancestors.

Taboo and Obsessional Neurosis

Freud states his thesis about the origin of guilt in two versions in *Totem and Taboo*. The first version comes after he has shown the similarity between taboo and obsessional neurosis. The second comes after he has treated totemism with similar insights from psychoanalytic observation. Thinking about taboo brings to the fore the existence of prohibitions against sexual intercourse with the father's women, and thinking about totemism brings to the fore prohibitions against killing the father. These are two parts of the Oedipus complex (as experienced by men). Having thus superimposed the analysis of neurotic male patients' conflicts upon primitive customs, Freud then added a concept of Darwin's, namely, that the earliest human society was characterized by a dominant male, plus subordinate juveniles unable to have access to females. The fully developed hypothesis of the origin of the incest taboo postulated a historical leap from this pattern of primate social organization to a higher level of civilization in which the young males, the father, and the women live in peace, a peace assured by the incest taboo but involving the inevitable oedipal conflict.

Let us now look more closely at Freud's thinking about taboo.

Freud's explanation of taboo uses the model of an obsessional's dread of touching. With his typical caution, he reminds us that the similarity between neurotic symptoms and taboo may be only superficial. The sense of guilt, however, is what is so remarkably similar in both. Both taboo and obsessional dread are "forcibly maintained by an irresistible fear. No external threat of punishment is required, for there is an internal certainty, a moral conviction that any violation will lead to intolerable disaster" (p. 27). Freud proceeds with an illuminating clinical example of the similarity between the obsessional symptoms of one of his patients and a taboo of a Maori chief. His comparison emphasizes the elements of contagion, as well as of "expiation, penance, defensive measures and purification" (p. 28), all obvious indicators of guilt.

In *Totem and Taboo* Freud's descriptive model for the development of an obsessional neurosis actually has emotional ambivalence as its centerpeice.

> Right at the beginning, in very early childhood, the patient shows a strong *desire* to touch [his own genitals]. This desire is promptly met by an *external* prohibition [which] is accepted since it finds support from powerful *internal* forces.

In a footnote he identifies this internal forces as stemming from "the child's loving relation to the authors of the prohibition," and goes on to say that the

> principal characteristic of the psychological constellation that becomes fixed in this way is the subject's *ambivalent* attitude. . . . He is constantly wishing to perform this act [of touching] and detests it as well. (p. 29, Freud's italics throughout)

To evade a theoretical formulation in which two powerful conflicting forces (emotions) are normally in conflict, Freud makes one of them (shame, desire) "unconscious," whereas the other (prohibition) is "noisily conscious." Thus he writes:

> The conflict between these two currents cannot be promptly settled because—there is no other way of putting it—they are localized in the subject's mind in such a manner that they cannot come up against each other. The prohibition is noisily conscious, while the persistent desire to touch is unconscious and the subject knows nothing of it. If it were not for this psychological factor, an ambivalence like this could neither last so long nor lead to such [neurotic] consequences. (pp. 29–30)

By thus making one part of the ambivalent constellation unconscious Freud translates the conflict into one between two "irrational" forces.

> As a result of the repression which has been enforced and which involves a loss of memory—an amnesia—the motives for the prohibition (which is conscious) remain unknown; and all attempts at disposing of it by intellectual processes must fail, since they cannot find any basis of attack. (p. 30)

But the translation of the conflict into one between unreasonable or senseless prohibition and "persistent" unconscious desire does not really evade a formulation of the conflict as between two powerful conflicting emotions. It merely transposes it into a conflict between two strong opposing "irrational" forces:

> The mutual inhibition of the two conflicting forces produces a need for dis-charge, for reducing the prevailing tension and to this may be attributed the performance of obsessive acts. . . . From one point of view they are evidence of remorse, efforts at expiation, and so on, while on the other hand they are substitutive acts to compensate the instinct for what has been prohibited. (p. 30)

Freud is now describing two equally powerful and conflicting emotional states, both of which are apparently irrational.

A difficulty thus arises from the fact that Freud is developing a model of normal guilt from a model of obsessional neurosis. If, in con-trast, ambivalent feelings of affection and hatred are regarded as normal in development, then their resolution by identification with the loved figures must issue in both guilt and shame.

When we come to Freud's application of his model of obsessional neurosis to the origin of the incest taboo, we find him ignoring the internal emotional supports for the acceptance of prohibition (guilt). For him the origin of guilt lies only in external prohibitions supplemented by "inherited" psychical traits.

> Taboos, we must suppose, are prohibitions of primeval antiquity which were at some time expertly imposed upon a generation of primitive men; they must, that is to say, no doubt have been impressed on them violently by a previous generation. These prohibitions must have concerned activities to-ward which there was a strong inclination. They must have persisted from generation to generation, perhaps merely as a result of tradition transmitted through parental and social authority. Possibly, however, in later genera-tions they may have become "organized" as an inherited psychical endow-ment. Who can decide whether such things as "innate ideas" exist, or whether in the present instance they have operated either alone or in con-junction with education, to bring about the permanent fixing of taboos?

Freud is here reduced to the same position he found so unacceptable in Wundt—a reliance on instinct for the origin of guilt.

Totemism and Phobia

Freud's second statement of the origin of guilt comes after he had made an extensive examination of contemporary studies of totemism. It was being widely studied at the time by many scholars, including Wundt, who regarded it as a transitional stage in the development of civilized religion.

Freud was impressed by Reinach's 12 articles of totemism—what

Freud calls a "catechism, as it were, of the totemic religion" (p. 101). These 12 articles are worth reproducing in full just as Freud lists them; their sense clearly implies nurturant and tender attitudes toward the totem animal, and protective attitudes expected from it, as well as the idea of common ancestry. Taken together, the 12 articles could be symbolically translated as representations of both parents, but Freud connects the totem symbol only with the father.

(1) Certain animals may neither be killed nor eaten, but individual members of the species are reared by human beings and cared for by them.

(2) An animal which has died an accidental death is mourned over and buried with the same honours as a member of the clan.

(3) In some instances the eating prohibition extends only to one particular part of the animal's body.

(4) When one of the animals which are usually spared has to be killed under the stress of necessity, apologies are offered to it and an attempt is made by means of various artifices and evasions to mitigate the violation of the taboo—that is to say, the murder.

(5) When the animal is made the victim of a ritual sacrifice, it is solemnly bewailed.

(6) On particularly solemn occasions and at religious ceremonies the skins of certain animals are worn. Where totemism is still in force, they are the totem animals.

(7) Clans and individuals adopt the names of animals—viz. of the totem animals.

(8) Many clans make use of representations of animals on their standards and weapons; the men have pictures of animals painted or tatooed on their bodies.

(9) If the totem is a formidable or dangerous animal, it is supposed to spare members of the clan named after it.

(10) The totem animal protects or gives warning to members of its clan.

(11) The totem animal foretells the future of the local members of its clan and serves them as guide.

(12) The members of the totemic clan often believe that they are related to the totem animal by a bond of a common ancestry.

In support of his interpretation that the totem animal symbolizes the father, Freud cites evidence from his and Ferenczi's analyses of young children—Hans, who was afraid of a horse, and (Ferenczi's) Arpad, who was so enamored of poultry birds that he cackled like them and was totally preoccupied with both caressing and torturing them. Freud takes note of the fact that Arpad's attitude toward the animal is positive whereas Hans's is negative, but quickly brings both cases into line as reflecting the Oedipus complex.

As was the case in his use of obsessional neurosis as the model for taboo, Freud's description of the dynamics of animal phobia clearly invokes ambivalent emotions as its centerpiece:

The hatred of the father that arises in a boy from rivalry for his mother is not able to achieve uninhibited sway over his mind; it has to contend against his old-established affection and admiration for the very same person. The child finds relief from the conflict arising out of this double-sided, this ambivalent emotional attitude toward his father by displacing his hostile and fearful feelings on to a *substitute* for his father. The displacement cannot, however, bring the conflict to an end, it cannot effect a clear-cut severance between the affectionate and hostile feelings. On the contrary, the conflict is resumed in relation to the object on which the displacement has been made: The ambivalence is extended to it. There could be little doubt that little Hans was not only *frightened* of horses; he also approached them with admiration and interest. As soon as his anxiety began to diminish, he identified himself with the dreaded creature; he began to jump about like a horse and in turn bit his father. At another stage in the resolution of his phobia, he did not hesitate to identify his parents with some other large animals. (p. 129, Freud's italics)

Freud seeks further confirmation of the equation he has made between totem and father by reviewing primitive customs or sacrifices. Here again he emphasizes that the sacrifice reflects an identification between the worshiper and his god. This is a positive emotional state of union, which also obtains between the child and the animal of which he is also afraid. It is a positive identification that keeps feelings ambivalent instead of unequivocally hostile. An extrapolation that follows—but that Freud does not explicitly make—is that positive identification is at the root of the state of guilt.

Having established to his own satisfaction the symbolic connection between the totem and the father, Freud proceeds to connect this "psychoanalytic translation" with "Darwin's theory of the earliest human society." This is Freud's second version of his hypothesis about the origin of guilt, and he sees its advantage as "establishing an unsuspected correlation between groups of phenomena that have hitherto been disconnected" (p. 141) (i.e., totemism, exogamy, and the incest taboo).

There is, of course, no place in the beginnings of totemism for Darwin's primal horde. All that we find there is a violent and jealous father who keeps all the females for himself and drives away his sons as they grow up. This earliest society has never been an object of observation. The most primitive kind of organization that actually comes across—and one that is in force today in certain tribes—consists of bands of males; these bands are composed of members with equal rights and are subject to the restrictions of the totemic system, including inheritance through the mother. Can this form of organization have developed out of the other? and if so along what lines?

If we call the celebration of the totem meal to our help, we shall be able to find an answer. One day the brothers who had been driven out came together, killed and devoured their father and so made an end of the patriarchal horde. [Freud footnotes the phrase "one day" by reminding his readers that "it would be foolish to aim at exactitude" in such questions as he is discussing.] United, they had the courage to do and succeeded in doing what would have been impossible for them individually. (Some cultural advance, perhaps command over some new weapon, had given them a sense of superior strength.) Cannibal savages as they were, it goes without saying that they devoured their victim as well as killing him. The violent primal father had doubtless been the feared and envied model of each one of the company of brothers; and in the act of devouring him they accomplished their identification with him, and each one acquired a portion of his strength. The totem meal, which is perhaps mankind's earliest festival, would thus be a repetition and a commemoration of this memorable and criminal deed, which was the beginning of so many things—of social organization, of moral restrictions and of religion.

In order that these latter consequences may seem plausible, leaving their premises on one side, we need only suppose that the tumultuous band of brothers was filled with the same contradictory feeling which we can see at work in the ambivalent father-complexes of our children and of our neurotic patients. They hated their father, who presented such a formidable obstacle to their craving for power; but they loved and admired him too. After they had got rid of him, had satisfied their hatred and had put into effect their wish to identify themselves with him, *the affection which had all this time been pushed under was bound to make itself felt. It did so in the form of remorse* [italics added]. A sense of guilt made its appearance, which in this instance coincided with the remorse felt by the whole group. The dead father became stronger than the living one had been—for events took the course we so often see them follow in human affairs today. What had up to then been prevented by his actual existence was thenceforward prohibited by the sons themselves in accordance with the psychological procedure so familiar to us in psychoanalysis under the name of "deferred obedience". They revoked their deed by forbidding the killing of the totem, the substitute for their father; and they renounced its fruits by resigning their claim to the women who had now been set free. Thus they created out of their filial sense of guilt the two fundamental taboos of totemism, which for that very reason inevitably corresponded to the two repressed wishes of the Oedipus complex. (pp. 141–143)

As the reader will see from this extensive quotation, Freud is actually in the tautological position of explaining the origin of guilt by assuming the existence of the sons' spontaneous feeling of guilt after parricide. He is in this position because he has no theory of human emotions as rooted in an attachment system. In his account, emotional states of violence, jealousy, courage, fear, envy, and identification are all taken for granted as natural phenomena in the primeval human being. Affection for the father is also included in the system of human emotions, although what the jealous and violent father has done to deserve it is not specified.

Freud is clearly "on the side" of the act of parricide, which made an end of the violent and jealous father who was oppressing his sons. He even speaks of it as made possible by some cultural advance, such as a new weapon. In Freud's view the sons' act of parricide was forward-looking and just. The women were also set free, as well as the sons. Freud also speaks of the primal deed as evoking a "creative sense of guilt" (p. 159).

Freud clearly describes the connection between affection and remorse or guilt. In his description the guilt arises out of two conflicting emotional states—affection and hatred, with affection being the immediate source. But Freud was so caught up in expounding the importance of the Oedipus complex as an explanatory principle in the formation of guilt that he simply passed over the problem of emotional ambivalence:

> I have often had occasion to point out that emotional ambivalence in the proper sense of the term—that is, the simultaneous existence of love and hate towards the same object—lies at the root of many important cultural institutions. We know nothing of the origin of this ambivalence. One possible assumption is that it is a fundamental phenomenon of our emotional life. But it seems to me to be quite worth considering another possibility, namely that originally it formed no part of our emotional life but was acquired by the human race in connection with their father-complex, precisely where the psychoanalytic examination of modern individuals finds it revealed at its strongest. (p. 157)

At this point Freud has a testy footnote in which he says that he is "used to being misunderstood," that he is "perfectly aware of the complexity of the phenomena under review," and that he "leaves to others the task of synthesizing the explanation into a unity." His difficulty in choosing ambivalence as a fundamental phenomenon of emotional life is well reflected in that footnote. As I have suggested throughout this book, the assumption, which Freud actually made in *Totem and Taboo* (as well as everywhere else), that ambivalence is a fundamental phenomenon of our emotional life has turned out to be a more fruitful path into new knowledge than has a strict version of the Oedipus complex.

THE DISJUNCTION BETWEEN FREUD AND PIAGET

Because Freud's concepts have been so contradictory, it has proved very difficult to formulate adequate empirical studies of the government or the functioning of morality under psychoanalytic guidance. Psychoanalytic studies of the influence of childrearing on subsequent morality have yielded mixed results (Fisher & Greenberg, 1977). As we shall see in the next chapter, cross-cultural studies have used broadly conceived Freudian concepts more fruitfully. One reason for the mixed findings in our own culture is the fact that Freudian theory has been interpreted by experimenters in a very strict oedipal sense, thus ignoring the central role of affectionate feelings in conscience formation that Freud's descriptions clearly implied. Thus, for example, Fisher and Greenberg (1977) formulate Freud's theory as predicting that the strength or severity of the male superego will be positively related to the punitive quality of the father. They cite Freud's (1928) statement in *Dostoievsky and Parricide* that the boy's superego is a direct function of the degree to which the father is hard, violent, and cruel. Empirical studies suggest that this proposition is not correct. A very careful study by Sears *et al.* (1965), for example, found no evidence that identification with the aggressor is a factor in the normal development of boys. Other studies have shown that the fathers of men with strong moral standards have not been strict with their sons; on the contrary, men with weak moral standards have had very punishing fathers. Thus in one study delinquent boys had had fathers who were significantly more punishing than those of a control group of nondeliquent boys (Bandura & Walters, 1959).[1]

In the context of this unhappy situation in psychoanalytic theory, Piaget's (1932) empirical study of moral judgment was eagerly adopted by academic psychologists as a starting point for further study. Although Piaget's work was narrowly confined to moral judgment, nor moral action or "moral sentiment," "cognitive-developmental" as well as "social learning" theorists found Piaget's statement of cognitive stages in moral judgment much more congenial than Freud's ambivalent reliance on conflicted passions. Kohlberg's translation of Piaget's work into an instrument measuring developmental stages of moral reasoning made possible a wealth of studies on moral action as well as moral judgment. But a disjunction was created between the two, as a result of which work on the cognitive and affective sides of the problem never seemed to mesh.

As has slowly become apparent, academic psychologists are beginning to sense that some very important affective components of both moral judgment and moral action have been neglected. Haan (1978) has shown experimentally that an "interpersonal formulation" of moral action produced more stable scores than Kohlberg's formal scores, especially when the "games" requiring ethical behavior were stressful. Haan's work was stimulated in part by the finding that adult American

[1]Although it is true that, in a footnote in *Civilization and Its Discontents* (1930), Freud specifically hypothesizes that delinquent children have been "brought up without love" (p. 130), on the very next page he is back to his one-sided version of the Oedipus complex.

women are more frequently rated as morally less mature than men on Kohlberg's scale. Haan argues that the

> moral reasoning of males who live in technological, rationalized societies, who reason at the level of formal operations and who defensively intellectualize and deny interpersonal and situational detail is especially favored in the Kohlberg scoring system. (p. 287)

As Blasi (1980) puts it in a recent literature review, what is needed is a focus on the "psychological nature of integrity, or of personal consistency, on the processes and skills that are involved in the capacity to invest one's life with meanings that are personally understood and accepted" (p. 40). One is reminded here of Freud's use of the more neutral term "meaning" to describe the fact that emotions were discernible in dreams. Blasi goes on to suggest (p. 41) that the neglect of "integrity" has resulted from the "overwhelming influence" of Piaget's rationalistic views of human nature, and he proposes that the "self" must be taken into account in theories of moral integrity, a statement that is close to identifying the neglected affective basis of morality.

Although Piaget has been criticized by Blasi and by psychoanalysts (e.g., Wolff, 1960) for his failure to consider the affective side of moral development, his theoretical statement very clearly implies that there is an affective basis for moral judgment. (Piaget, it is true, cites Bovet, not Freud, as his mentor.) Piaget ascribes the genesis of the feeling of moral obligation, first, to the child's acceptance of commands from "someone whom he respects." Moreover, he clearly bases this statement on an affective basis for morality on "Durkheim's doctrine of the social genesis of respect and morality" (p. 44). Piaget simply expands Durkheim's doctrine to include a concept of "mutual respect" as the adult basis for morality. He implies that the transition from unilateral respect, in which external authority is "sacred," to mutual respect, in which the feeling of equality prevails, is the transition from childhood to adult morality. Piaget, in fact, eloquently contrasts two moralities on the basis of their affective content.

> The ethics of authority, which is of duty and obedience, leads . . . to the confusion of what is just with the content of established law and the acceptance of expiatory punishment. The ethics of mutual respect, which is that of good (as opposed to duty) and of autonomy, leads to the development of equality, which is the idea at the bottom of distributive justice and reciprocity. *Solidarity between equals* appears once more as the source of a whole set of complementary and coherent moral ideas which characterize the rational mentality. (p. 324, italics added)

Piaget regards the affective task behind the development of morality to be the "personal cultivation of solidarity" (p. 345). Although the language they use is very different, Piaget's emphasis on "solidarity" as the basis for a developed morality is not unlike Freud's emphasis on "identification." Both are "social" emotions (as well as cognitive states) that keep people attached to each other.

In a review of research on moral internalization, Hoffman (1977) finds that the use of empathy—that is, induction in the child of the state of mind of the "other"—is correlated with a high level of morality. Although the studies he reviews are—lamentably—only correlational for the most part, they show that "power assertion" on the parents' part is correlated with "fear of detection," and that "love withdrawal" is associated with "inhibition of anger." Hoffman's review also suggests that during the first year of a child's life 90% of the mother–child interactions are affectionate. During the second year, 60% of the interactions are aimed at obtaining the child's obedience. This evidence also suggests that obedience follows an earlier period of affectionate connection (Hogan, 1975). These findings are all consonant with Freud's description of the affectionate basis of morality, but not with his oedipal theory.

CHAPTER 9

Psychoanalysis in Cross-Cultural Perspective
The Problem of Human Nature

Just before World War I, Durkheim and Freud each independently proposed that guilt is an internalization of cultural values. Since then, the
field of personality and culture has burgeoned into its now massive
proportions. Interdisciplinary studies, involving psychology, sociology,
and anthropology, have developed into what is now the field of psychoanalytic anthropology.

It was Talcott Parsons (1964) who called attention to the remarkable
convergence of thought between Freud and Durkheim. In particular,
Parsons was impressed by Freud's idea that each new ego is formed out
of cathexes abandoned by the id. As Parsons interprets this idea, a very
early identification with significant others forms the basis for the internalization of culture; and it was thus that Freud's concept of identification fostered the integration of psychology, sociology, and anthropology
(Parsons, 1958). Major anthropologists, such as Margaret Mead and
Ruth Benedict, have also acknowledged Freud's influence. Through
popularization of their work, Freud's description of the affectional basis
for an individual's socialization became a part of the accepted scientific
wisdom.

In this chapter we shall examine some of the many controversies
generated by Freud's writings on the origin of guilt, controversies that

have contributed to the growth of the field of personality and culture. Freud's view, as narrowly interpreted by Roheim (1945), was that culture itself is a "defense" against anxiety. Similarly, orthodox psychoanalysts (e.g., Jones, 1924/1964) insisted that the Oedipus complex was a human universal regardless of prevailing social and economic conditions. These narrow interpretations gave ammunition to critics of psychoanalysis for its neglect of the rational side of human morality. Thus both Piaget and Lévi-Strauss, sharing the same French rationalistic tradition, became identified as anti-Freudians.

From a different viewpoint, Freud's studied neglect of social and economic conditions surrounding morality became the target of the psychoanalytic revisionists: Adler, Horney, Fromm, and Reich. All of these critics attempted to integrate Freud's insights about primary process with the stress created on human beings by economic and social oppression and war. A related controversy devloped over Freud's androcentric views, beginning with Horney and continuing into present-day feminist scholarship. Thus, as we shall see in this chapter, ideas have progressed from Freud's pioneering study of hysterical women, whose denigrated status in the family he acknowledged but did not pursue, to recent feminist critiques of a male-centered model of morality (Haan; 1978; Lewis, 1978; Gilligan, 1981). This contemporary focus on Freud's androcentrism highlights his theoretical neglect of the human attachment emotions.

Roheim, Malinowski, and Orthodox Freudianism

One of the earliest psychoanalytic anthropologists, Geza Roheim (1945), revisited the Australian Arunta people who figured so heavily in Frazer's work and thus in Freud's *Totem and Taboo*.[1] Roheim adopted a Freudian view that the common denominator of all human cultures, whatever their political and social structure, is that they are a defense against anxiety. Anxiety itself is a universal product of the Oedipus complex. It is primarily guilt anxiety arising out of the underlying aggression that human culture only minimally curtails. Thus Roheim writes: "Religion and society are erected as walls of defense against libidinal dangers inherent in the infantile situation" (1945, p. 176). Ad-

---

[1]Roheim's film of the subincision rites practiced on the penis of adolescent initiates has been widely used in laboratory studies—for example, by Lazarus and coworkers in their studies on the psychophysiology of emotions, and by Witkin, Goodenough, and myself in our studies of the incorporation of presleep stress stimuli into dreams.

hering to a strict Freudian conception, Roheim interpreted the complicated initiation rites practiced by the Arunta and other Australian groups as well as their dreams. The Arunta are a prime example of a patriarchal society. In a matriarchal society, oedipal dynamics were not quite so powerful an interpretive tool, as Malinowski (1927) discovered.

One of the most illuminating (and amusing) controversies in psychoanalytic anthropology occurred in the 1920s when Malinowski set out to test Freud's concept of a universal Oedipus complex (A. Parsons, 1964). On the basis of fieldwork in the matriarchal Trobriand Islands, Malinowski drew the conclusion that the Oedipus complex was not universal, being only one of a number of possible "nuclear complexes." In the matriarchal family Malinowski observed that a triangular relationship existed among brother, sister, and sister's son. A boy is subject to the authority of his maternal uncle rather than that of his biological father. Even though Malinowski emphasized that the ambivalent feelings between a boy and his maternal uncle were quite similar to the ambivalent feelings in a patriarchal triangle, and even though Malinowski thus made psychological sense out of a stringent, "supreme" incest taboo between brother and sister, including complicated brother–sister avoidance rituals, Ernest Jones, speaking for establishment psychoanalysis in 1924, was still not satisfied with anything less than a view that the Oedipus complex as described by Freud is universal.

Jones went so far as to interpret matriarchal society itself as a "denial" of primordial father–son ambivalence, and to insist that father–son ambivalence must be present in Trobriand society at least in infancy. A good deal of Jones's fire was directed at Malinowski's observation that the biological paternity of the father is not acknowledged in Trobriand official beliefs, although Malinowski also presented data to show that the Trobrianders were actually well acquainted with the biological facts of reproduction. Jones interpreted Trobriand beliefs about paternity as a "spirit entering the womb" as a "denial" of the early ambivalent affects between father and son, an interpretation that Malinowski's data simply controverted: The relationships between father and son in Trobriand society are actually very close and affectionate from infancy onward.

This controversy, in retrospect, is an indication of the difficulties encountered when emotional relationships—ambivalent feelings in particular—are not considered of sufficient theoretical status to be prime movers of psychological events. It also reflects the difficulty in focusing on one set of emotions—aggression arising in a nuclear patriarchal family. Most important of all, the controversy illuminates Freud's refusal to consider the impact of the material conditions of existence on family dynamics.

LÉVI-STRAUSS: AN ANTI-FREUDIAN ANTHROPOLOGIST?

One of the severest ciritics of psychoanalytic anthroplogy is Lévi-Strauss. Nevertheless, his basic approach to anthroplogy bears some remarkable similarities to Freud's. Thus Lévi-Strauss considers that the anthropologist's task is to "grasp the unconscious structures underlying each institution and each custom, in order to obtain a principle of interpretation valid for other institutions and customs" (1967, p. 22). This is precisely what Freud undertook to do in his interpretation of the variety of totem and taboo customs. Lévi-Strauss assumes, moreover, that "forms are fundamentally the same for all minds—ancient and modern, primitive and civilized" (p. 21). Freud also assumed the fundamental unity of psychological processes in human beings (although he also contradicted his own assumption. In *Totem and Taboo* he wrote:

> Psychoanalysis has shown us that everyone possesses in his unconscious mental activity an apparatus which enables him to interpret other people's reactions, that is, to undo the distortions which other people have imposed on the expression of their feelings. (1913, p. 159)

What Freud is saying here is that emotions can be universally apprehended.

Ironically, the point where he overtly parts company with Freud is over what Lévi-Strauss regards as Freud's overreliance on affectivity. Lévi-Strauss distrusts affectivity as the "most obscure side of man," specifically contradicting Freud's theory as follows:

> Contrary to what Freud maintained, social constraints, whether positive or negative, cannot be explained, either in their origin or in their persistence, as the effects of impulses or emotions which appear again and again, with the same characteristics and during the course of centuries and millennia in different individuals. (1962/1969, p. 140)

The issue, as Lévi-Strauss poses it, is thus the power of emotions to explain or govern social institutions. As we have seen, this is precisely the issue of anchoring emotions in "reality" that gave Freud so much difficulty both in *Totem and Taboo* (1913) and in *Inhibitions, Symptoms and Anxiety* (1926).

The theoretical difficulties at issue here are well illustrated in differing interpretations placed by Lévi-Strauss (1968) and Roheim (1945) upon the same primitive creation myth. The myth of the Wawilak sisters, reported by Lloyd Warner, comes from the Australian Murngin people, who practice subincision rites very similar to the Arunta rites that Roheim photographed. This creation myth is of particular interest because it locates the origin of cultures in an act of incest. Lévi-Strauss analyzes the myth of the Wawilak sisters as an expression of the rationally perceived contradiction between men's social power and women's natural fertility. (He stops short of calling the perceived contradiction an injustice.) Roheim analyzes the myth as reflecting man's castration anxiety transformed into a self-protecting identification with the menstruating woman, an identification that is accomplished by slitting the penis of the initiates.

Let us look more closely at the details of the myth of the Wawilak sisters. (The text presented here is taken from Lévi-Strauss [1968] but Roheim's account of the myth does not differ significantly.)

> At the beginning of time the Wawilak sisters set off on foot towards the sea, naming places, animals and plants as they went. One of them was pregnant and the other carried her child. Before their departure they had both indeed had incestuous relations with men of their own moiety [kinship group].
> After the birth of the younger sister's child, they continued their journey and one day stopped near a water hole where the great snake Yurlunggur lived who was the totem of the Dua moiety to which the sisters belonged. The older sister polluted the water with menstrual blood. The outraged python came out, causing a deluge of rain and a general flood and then swallowed the women and their children. When the snake raised himself the waters covered the entire earth and its vegetation. When he lay down again the flood receded. . . . Had the Wawilak sisters not committed incest and polluted the water hole of Yurlunggur there would have been neither life nor death, neither copulation nor reproduction on the earth, and there would have been no cycle of seasons.

Lévi-Strauss's interpretation of this myth rests on a number of conditions prevailing in Murngin life. First, they live in an area of the world where there is a rainy season and a dry season, and this seasonal change is so regular that it can be predicted almost to the day. (Lévi-Strauss observes that the graph of rainfall recorded at Port Darwin over a period of 46 years might be thought of as depicting a picture of the snake, Yurlunggur.) The rainy season causes the Murngin people to disperse and take refuge in small groups; during the rainy season they are also threatened with famine. A few days after the flood recedes, vegetation is lush and animals reappear. The rainy season is thus the bad season; the dry season is the good season.

Second, this Australian group shares with others of its neighborhood a system in which old men enjoy sexual privileges, and they also control esoteric and cruel initiation rites to which the young men in the tribe must submit. Women are excluded from these rites; women and young men are in a position of inferior social power in this and many other ways.

Lévi-Strauss's explanation of the Murngin creation myth is that it establishes "homologies between natural and social conditions." These equivalencies are put together in order to manage contradictions in a reasonable way.

First, there is a homology between the snake and the rainy season. Both the snake and the rainy season are equated with maleness. The Murngin consciously associate the snake and the rainy season on the basis that the rainy season is the fertilizing period; the snake is the (male) fertilizing agent. (Although Lévi-Strauss does not mention it, this concept fits Freudian theory, in which the snake is the symbol of the phallus.) The "protagonists" of the great mythical drama, the snake and the Wawilak sisters, are associated with the rainy and the dry seasons, respectively. The former represents the male and the initiated, the latter the female and the uninitiated. The equivalences are roughly the following:

Pure, sacred; male, superior, fertilizing (rains), bad season
Impure, profane; female, inferior, fertilized (land), good season

The contradiction embedded in these equivalences is the equation of the bad season with the pure, sacred, superior, fertilizing male. On the natural plane, the good season is clearly superior to the bad; on the social plane, the good season is made inferior. The problem becomes how to interpret the contradiction. If the good season is said to be superior and male, then both social power and sterility would have to be attributed to the female element. This "absurdity" is disguised by making "a double division of the whole society into two classes of men and women (now ritually as well as sexually differentiated)." The young men are classed with the women and made inferior to the old men. And

> in consequence men forgo embodying the happy side of existence for they cannot both rule and personify it. Irrevocably committed to the role of gloomy owners of a happiness accessible to them only through an intermediary, they fashion an image of themselves on the model of their sages and old men [and] to attain full masculinity young men must . . . lastingly submit [to severe initiation rites at puberty.] (p. 94)

Lévi-Strauss's interpretation thus follows the rational processes by which a people make sense of the conditions they find around them. The myth, and the initiation rites for which it is the basis, help to make sense of and to perpetuate the inferior social position of young men and of women, which the culture recognizes as a contradiction, if not as an injustice.

In contrast, Roheim analyzes the myth as evolving out of the mystery for the little boy of his separation from his mother.

> He was separated from the mother when she was copulating with his father and when she was menstruating; now in the mysteries *he* represents the primal scene and a menstruating woman. The sight of the menstrual blood calls forth castration anxiety in the men, society is built up on an inversion of this anxiety, for it is the men who are bleeding [in the initiation rites] and the women who must not catch sight of the "menstrual blood" of the [subincised] males. The men who might be weakened by the blood of the women now fortify each other by the blood of the fathers. (p. 176)

What Roheim's interpretation omits is the connection between the content of the creation myth and such material considerations surrounding Murngin life as the rainy and dry seasons. But when Lévi-Strauss and Roheim address family dynamics, a comparison of their interpretations yields many similarities. The former, for example, simply takes for granted the symbolic equation of the snake and the phallus. He also tells us that there is a "very profound analogy which people throughout the world seem to find between copulation and eating." He explains that the "lowest common denominator of the union of the sexes and the union of the eater and the eaten is that they both effect a conjunction by complementarity." He observes further that

> the equation of male with devourer and female with the devoured is more familiar to us and certainly the more prevalent in the world, but one must not forget that the inverse equivalence is often found at a mythological level in the theme of the vagina dentata. (p. 106)

As we see, Lévi-Strauss emphasizes the rational basis for the simile between eating and intercourse; Freud and Roheim would emphasize the affective foundation for the simile in the pleasurable memories and feelings of suckling at the breast, memories that are revived during intercourse. Lévi-Strauss's idea that the men "fashion an image of themselves" on the model of their sages and lastingly submit to cruel initiation rites is really not too different from Roheim's concept of defensive identification. Moreover, the concept that the myth and the initiation rites are *justifications* for men's superior social power is embedded in both Lévi-Strauss's and Roheim's interpretations. Both make use of Freudian "primary-process" transformations of conflicted or ambivalent feelings in making their interpretive leaps.

Lévi-Strauss, Roheim, and Freud all also share a strong androcentric bias. Lévi-Strauss's famous theory of the origin of the incest taboo pictures this shift from nature to culture as occurring through the men in differing kinship groups exchanging their women as "gifts."

> The prohibition of incest is less a rule prohibiting marriage with the mother, sister or daughter, than a rule obliging the mother, sister or daughter to be

> given to others. It is the supreme rule of the gift, and it is clearly this aspect, too often unrecognized, which allows its nature to be understood. (1949)

It is taken for granted in this account, and by Roheim and Freud as well, that men are in the position of ownership of their women. Only recently, as an outgrowth of an amalgam between feminist scholarship and Freudian revisionism, has this fundamental assumption been questioned (G. Rubin, 1975).

FREUD AND MARXISM

As suggested earlier, Freud's insistence on the historical reality of the primal deed was a form of adherence to a materialist tradition in which psychological events, especially emotional ones, were epiphenomena of physical events occurring in the "real world." In this respect, Freud was adopting a position quite similar to that of the Marxist critics of civilized morality, who also saw the origin of morality in the "real" conditions of existence, what Marx called "praxis." What divided Freud from the Marxists was the aspect of reality on which they chose to concentrate. Freud concentrated on the conditions under which the species reproduced itself, and in this choice inevitably focused more on the organization of the reproducing family than on the background economic conditions. Marx saw the origin of morality in a larger "praxis"— that is, in the practical conditions of economic life necessary for survival, as well as the conditions governing the species's sexual relations. Engels, for example, introduces his book on the origin of the family as follows:

> According to the materialist conception, the decisive factor in history is, in the last resort, the production and reproduction of immediate life. But this itself is of a twofold character. On the one hand, the production of the means of subsistence, of food, clothing and shelter and the tools requisite thereto; on the other, the production of human beings themselves, the propagation of the species. (1884, p. 5)

Actually, both Freud and the Marxists identified exploitation as a condition of human existence within which morality was born. Freud clearly perceived that the father's treatment of his sons was unjust and that their act of rebellion was creative. Marx and Engels perceived that economic exploitativeness had been a steady feature of human life since the start of civilization, and that civilized morality is flawed to the extent that it fosters submission to exploitative rulers.

The issue over which Freud and the Marxists remain divided is the origin of exploitativeness. Freud saw its origins in the inevitable circumstances of our primate ancestry, which required a dominant male for species survival and healthful exogamous matings. Marx and Engels saw the origin of exploitativeness as a concomitant of historical development from primitive economic conditions to more advanced technological conditions. In Freud's view exploitativeness is inherent in human (sexual) nature along with the violence that justly opposed it and was then transformed into guilt. Each new infant is essentially selfish (narcissistic), that is, amoral. In the Marxist view, exploitativeness is not inherent in human nature, but only in civilized human beings, whose morality has been deformed by the conditions of their economic existence. In Freud's view, civilization and morality have jointly advanced over primitive sexual selfishness; in the Marxist view established morality has declined as civilization has advanced.

It is instructive to contrast Engels's prehistoric model of humanity with Freud's. In the former, prehistoric society was characterized by communal ownership of the means of subsistence and a marriage and family structure that was similarly communal. "Group marriage, the form in which whole groups of men and whole groups of women belong to one another and which leaves little scope for jealousy" (1884, p. 30) was then in existence. This earliest form of family life originally included incestuous matings; "natural selection," however, dictated that the incest taboo should be instituted first between parents and children, then between sisters and brothers, and then in a widening circle of kinship groups. Engels's model of prehistoric family life is thus the opposite of Freud's bloody domination by the male. "Incestuous" matings become troublesome only on hygienic grounds; once this happens, however, the absolutely peaceful conditions of group marriage are replaced by an ever-widening circle of restrictions on mating until there develops a "scarcity of (eligible) women" (p. 40). Women thereafter are obtained either by purchase or by capture. (It should be noted at this point that Engels is just as androcentric as Freud. Incest regulations could equally well have been supposed to result in a scarcity of eligible men as of women.)

The decline of this peaceful communal family proceeds *pari passu* with a change from communal ownership of the means of subsistence to individual ownership of the means of production. This development accompanies the division of labor, the acquisition of herds, the development of tools and weapons, and the individual ownership of land. With these developments comes exploitative behavior, both economically and in sexual relationships. Civilization's achievements have occurred as a result of setting in motion the lowest instincts and passions in man and developing them at the expense of all his other abilities. From its first day to this, greed was the driving spirit of civilization, wealth and again wealth and once more wealth, wealth not only of society but of the single scurvy individual—here was its one and final aim. (p. 145)

In Engels's model, the development of incest taboos was not the source of guilt. Moreover, prehistoric humanity was, by implication, both peaceable and guilt-free. Division of labor was originally equal between the sexes, as was power between them.

> The man fights in the war, goes hunting and fishing and procures the raw material of food and the tools necessary for doing so. The woman looks after the house and the preparation of the food and clothing, cooks, weaves and sews. Each is the owner of the instruments he or she makes and uses: the man of the weapons, the hunting and fishing implements, the woman of the household gear. Under condition of equality of ownership and in the mastery of tasks there is equality between the sexes. (p. 131)

It is amusing to note in passing how taken for granted are stereotyped ideas of men's and women's occupations. Even Engels, writing a treatise that aims at the liberation of women, imagines his mythical peaceable savage to be a warrior and hunter, whereas Ms. peaceable savage, although equal in rank, still minds the house. But Engels's account, unlike Freud's, assumes that the oppression of women, like the oppression of men, derived mainly from the circumstances of economic life.

It is instructive to realize that Engels's model of primitive humanity was based on the revolutionary model that Rousseau elaborated a century earlier. In that model the chief characteristic of humanity before civilization is *pitie*, that is, compassion. In his *Essay on the Origin and Foundations of Inequality among Men* (1964), Rousseau tells us that as he first began to study this question he saw "only the violence of the powerful and the oppression of the weak" (p. 97).

> Throwing aside . . . scientific books, which only teach us how to see men such as they have made each other, and meditating on the first and simplest operations of the human soul, I believe I discover there two principles which are anterior to reason. One of them pushes us forcibly to consider our own well-being and our own survival, and the other inspires in us a natural repugnance towards seeing any sentient being, and especially our fellow-men, either perish or suffer. (p. 95)

To this second principle Rousseau gives the name *pitie*. *Pitie* he defines as a "natural sentiment which by moderating the love of self in each individual leads to the mutual preservation of the whole species" (p. 100). As Rousseau conceived of *pitie*, it is the characteristic of primitive human beings that was suppressed or cut off by the development of civilization. Primitive human beings, seeing another person suffer, identify with that suffering and want to help. In civilized society, one human being sees another suffer and is indifferent; unconcern is codified by laws that distinguish human beings according to rank or wealth, and the unconcern is thus granted moral justification. Compassion is no longer required of human beings because some people have been rationally discriminated against as different and inferior. In this sense, civilization is built on a deformation of human nature, the loss of human capacity for *pitie*.

It is worth noting that Freud's descriptive account of the origin of civilization is not too different from Rousseau's in emphasizng the fundamental importance of identification or compassion. It is only in his more theoretical formulations that Freud neglects compassion.

Freud's view of human nature, as he continued to express it in his later writings, varied between occasional statements suggesting a view of human nature as fundamentally social and an opposite view of people as basically lazy and aggressive. Thus in *Group Psychology and the Analysis of the Ego* (1921) Freud writes that it is

> only rarely and under certain exceptional conditions [that] individual psychology [is] in a position to disregard the relations of [an] individual to others. In the individual's mental life someone else is invariably involved, as a model, as an object, as a helper, as an opponent; and so from the very first individual psychology, in this extended but entirely justifiable sense of the words, is at the same time social psychology as well. (p. 69)

In *The Future of an Illusion* (1927a) he voices the opposite view—namely, that "every individual is virtually an enemy of civilization" (p. 6). He goes on to say that "there are present in all men destructive and therefore anti-social and anti-cultural trends and . . . in a great number of people these are strong enough to determine their behavior in society" (p. 7). Freud considers whether an equitable distribution of wealth would not make the burden of civilization easier. He quickly concludes to the contrary, justifying his answer by reference to the nature of the masses. "It is just as impossible to do without coercion of the masses by a minority as it is to dispense with coercion in the work of civilization. For masses are lazy and unintelligent; they have no love for instinctual renunciation. . . ." It is clear, moreover, that Freud is specifically responding negatively to Marxist views: Although he does not identify these by name, he does make explicit reference to the "great experiment in progress in the vast country that stretches between Europe and Asia" (p. 9); and although he has just described the masses as needing coercion by a minority, he maintains that he is not making judgments on the feasibility of socialism. In *Civilization and Its Discontents* (1930) Freud is even more explicit in asserting that socialism is based on "psychological premises [that are] an untenable illusion. In abolishing private property we deprive human love of aggression of one of its instruments" (p. 113).

Adler, Fromm, and Reich were all critics within the psychoanalytic movement who took Freud to task for his neglect of social and economic considerations. Their work arose out of the revolutionary and socialist tradition that Freud specifically disavowed. They focused on connecting political and social conditions of oppression within Western culture with the individual's neurotic guilt, via the distortions of the family into a transmission belt for exploitative and patriarchal values that conflict with the family's nurturant functions. This line of thinking characterized Western culture as "sick."

One of the most trenchant and compelling criticisms of Freud's views on guilt is found in Erich Fromm's work. What Freud neglected, in Fromm's view, was the realization that the family is the instrument for creating a socially acceptable character modeled on the image of societal values, not just in the image of the father's values. The father is not the prototype (*Vorbild*) of social authority but its replica (*Abbild*). In *Escape from Freedom* (1941), Fromm introduced the concept of "social character . . . molded by the mode of existence of a given society" and in turn helping to shape the "social process" (pp. 296–297).

In later works, particularly in *The Sane Society* (1955), Fromm describes how bourgeois capitalism fosters a human being who is "competitive, hoarding, exploitative, authoritarian, aggressive and individualistic" (p. 99). Fromm accepts Freud's view that emphasis on strict anal toilet training would be the familial transmission route for these characteristics. But he broadens Freud's clinical description of the anal (sexual) impulses and their regulation into a description of a bourgeois character that is derived from and congruent with the requirements of life under competitive capitalism. Thus Fromm interpreted the rise of Protestant individualistic ethics—involving both the freedom and the isolation of the individual—as a result of the collapse of medieval feudalism. Individual feelings of powerless isolation and doubt were responsible for the appeal of Luther's and Calvin's doctrines of original sin. These doctrines "stabilized the characterological changes and in turn became productive forces in the development of capitalism" (1941, p. 297).

In a similar spirit of broadening Freud's concepts to include economic and social forces, Reich (1971) interpreted the success of fascist values in Germany and Italy. Specifically, he traced the mystical appeal of fascist slogans—"honor," "duty," "sacred motherhood," "purification of German blood," and "masochism"—to psychic defenses against sadism. Sadism and masochism are fostered by the constraints of monopoly capitalism on the helpless individual. Thus Reich interpreted the ecstatic feeling of exalted virtue that characterized fascist crowd behavior as transformed yearnings arising out of sexual defenses. Reich also commented on the "frequent cohesion of sadistic brutality and mystical sentiment" in war leaders throughout history (1971, p. 148).

An amalgam of Freudian revisionist views, incorporating in particular many of Fromm's concepts, comprised the set of conceptual tools with which psychoanalytic anthropologists of the 1930s began to work. An early collaborative effort between an anthropologist and an psychoanalyst, Cora DuBois and Abram Kardiner, was a study of the people of Alor (DuBois, 1944). This study focused on the "modal personality" evolving out of the press of socioeconomic forces on childrearing practices. A relatively high degree of feeding deprivation was observed in Alorese infants as a result of their mother's responsibility for the maintenance of the subsistence economy. The emotional dynamics evoked by the pattern of early oral deprivation, in combination with sexual permissiveness, resulted in a "modal personality" described as anxious, suspicious, lacking in self-esteem, and varying between feelings of helplessness and grandiosity. The study boldly used Western measuring instruments such as the Rorschach, Word Association, Children's Drawings, and the Porteus Maze on the questionable assumption that those instruments are "culture free"; its methodological rigor is therefore not of the highest. But the study related the oppressive economic conditions of Alorese women to their childrearing practices and attitudes in a way that foreshadows recent feminist scholarship.

Cross-cultural studies of socialization have also made use of the technique of comparing childrearing practices in widely different cultures. An early study making use of this method is that of Whiting and Child (1953), who made use of correlational methods to test hypotheses about the relation of culture to personality. Their formulations resulted from an integration of psychoanalytic and behavioral concepts (Dollard, Doob, Miller, Mowrer, & Sears, 1939). Whiting and Child were particularly impressed by Freud's concept that identification is the process by which guilt is internalized. They went on, however, to reformulate Freud's notion in terms of general behavior theory. This combined formulation suggests that the child "imitates the evaluative responses of his parents and thus punishes himself [by guilt feelings] whenever he has done something for which he believes his parents feel he should be punished" (p. 227). Whiting and Child used the extent to which a person who gets sick blames himself for getting sick as a cultural "index of responsibility," that is, of the internalization of guilt. They correlated this index against such socialization practices as weaning and toilet training in 35 different societies. They interpreted their findings as offering some tentative support for the process of socialization through identification.

Perhaps the most far-reaching development in this area has been Berry's (1976) ecological-cultural-behavioral model for conceptualizing the basis of childrearing practices and predicting their consequences in an individual's cognitive style. Berry's model combines Freudian concepts with Witkin's. Building on the evidence obtained by Barry, Child, and Bacon (1959) to the effect that food accumulation modes are related to such child-training variables as responsibility, obedience, nurturance, achievement, self-reliance, and independence, Berry hypothesized that field dependence is related to training for obedience. The overt role of Freudian thinking in this study is muted, but both the concept of childrearing practices and the concept of field dependence as a personality variable are outgrowths of Freudian thinking.

FEMINISM AND FREUDIAN REVISIONISTS

Perhaps the most promising modern development has been the growth of an amalgam of feminist thinking with Freudian insights into the emotional implications of social and economic conditions for family dynamics (Chodorow, 1978; Lewis, 1976; Mitchell, 1974). This amalgam, focused on the broad question of women's widespread cross-cultural social inferiority, has documented the ill effects of this lopsided distribution of power between the sexes, using Freudian insights into the "primary-process" transformations of ambivalent feelings.

I have elsewhere developed in detail the thesis that an exploitative society pushes men and women into internalizing its values differently (Lewis, 1976). Women are more prone to experiencing their superego as shame, whereas men are more prone to guilt. (This route of understanding sex differences in mental illness is also a major theme of Volume 1.)

One important focus of attention has been on the consequences of the fact that women bear and nurture children but are at the same time so often economic and social inferiors. In particular, the effects of cross-sex first caretaker for men and same-sex first caretaker for women have been studied in interaction with male power. Chodorow (1971), for example, theorizes about cross-sex rearing for men as follows: For children of both sexes, the earliest identity is feminine since they are reared by women who are the providers of food. The "primary-optative" identity is feminine for both sexes. But as boys grow up, especially in father-dominant cultures, they become aware of male power and therefore aware that a secondary "operative" identity is needed. This helps to account for the cross-cultural finding that male initiation rites tend to occur more often in patrilocal societies. The function of these rites, especially in father-absent societies, is to "brainwash the primary optative feminine identity and establish firmly the secondary male identity" (Burton & Whiting, 1961, p. 90). One cross-cultural study showed, in fact, that male violence is greatest in cultures (as in the Indian caste system) where the husband and wife are forbidden to sleep together, eat together, work or play together (B. Whiting, cited in Chodorow, 1971). Another cross-cultural study showed that male narcissism is prevalent in societies where there is greater emotional distance between husband and wife than between mother and child (Slater & Slater, 1965). Clearly, these studies make use of Freud's concepts but take them as restricted to patriarchal societies that oppress women.

Chodorow's study (1978) of the reproduction of mothering is an excellent example of the amalgam of Freudian-revisionist and feminist thinking. Chodorow suggests that "contemporary reproduction of mothering occurs through socially structured psychological processes." She uses psychoanalytic thinking to unravel these processes.

> Women, as mothers, produce daughters with mothering capacities and the desire to mother. . . . By contrast, women as mothers (and men as not-mothers) produce some whose nurturant capacities and needs have been systematically curtailed and repressed. (p. 7)

Chodorow's study offers a powerful set of arguments for the beneficial effects of "parenting," that is, full participation of both sexes in child-rearing.

Another important study of the psychological consequences of sexual inequality is Herman's (1981) work on father–daughter incest. Specifically, evidence has now accumulated showing that father–daughter incest occurs much more often than mother–son incest. This difference is, in turn, an understandable outcome of patriarchal power, which fosters the attitude that women are possessions of men and thus "justifies" incest with their daughters. If, in addition, men do not participate in the (socially inferior) task of childrearing, their capacity for affectionate and empathic feeling with their children is diminished, and their ethical judgment about incest is grossly impaired. As Herman puts it:

> The structure of the patriarchal family, in which child care is relegated to subordinate women, determines that men and women internalize the taboo very differently. In a family where fathers rule and mothers nurture, the most strictly observed incest taboo must be the prohibition on sexual rela-

tions between mother and son; the most frequently broken taboo must be that on relations between father and daughter. (p. 58)

Gilligan (1983) has persuasively argued that the social sciences do not have an adequate theory of moral development because of their androcentric bias. In this criticism, which is specifically directed against Piaget and Kohlberg, Freud and Lévi-Strauss may also appropriately be included. Gilligan points out that Piaget took boys' moral development as his model, as did Kohlberg. Gilligan contrasts the "ethic of care," which women often voice in solving moral dilemmas, with the "ethic of responsibility," more often voiced by men. As she puts it: "The ethic of care restores the concept of love to the moral domain, uniting cognition and affect by tying reflection to the experience of relationship" (p. 45).

Epilogue

An observer of the history of ideas might have expected that, immediately following Freud's demonstration of the role of the moral emotions of shame and guilt in both abnormal and normal behavior, research into the psychology of emotions should have burgeoned. On the contrary, during the nearly hundred years since *Studies on Hysteria* (Breuer & Freud, 1893–1895) the psychology of emotions has remained (in spite of numerous exceptions) a somewhat isolated area of inquiry both in academia and in psychoanalysis itself. Moreover, so far as I know, *Freud and Modern Psychology* is unique in proposing that emotions cannot be understood apart from their place within the human affectional attachment system. Although many observers have acknowledged the social function of emotions, inquiry has focused on the single individual, rather than on the emotional attachment system in which each person is embedded throughout his or her entire lifetime.

One reason for the relative neglect of emotions in psychology, in spite of Freud's observations, was Freud's own choice of a theoretical system in which to place his observations. In Volume 1 I demonstrated that Freud's theoretical system, although explicitly psychological, was modeled after physiological processes of impulse arousal and discharge. Freud was thus attempting to fit complicated social and emotional transactions between people into a narrow intrapsychic framework. Today's biochemists tell us that we must distinguish carefully between schizophrenia, which involves the stress of social interaction, and depression, which involves the stress of social loss. That different neuroregulators are involved in the different emotional patterns clearly points to the centrality of the affectional ties that are threatened in both disorders. Freud was the first to describe a different pattern of withdrawal of libido in schizophrenia and depression.

Out of his background as an experimental neurologist Freud formulated a theoretical system of behavior based not on emotions or social
connectedness, but on the existence of unknown or unconscious sources
of energy—instincts—which seek the pleasure of discharge (after the
manner of nerve impulses) but are blocked by counterforces, also originating in instincts. So, for example, he used the terms "quota of affect"
and "sum of excitations" interchangeably to describe how affect "covers" the surface of experience as if it were an "electric charge." Paradoxically, although a "quota of affect" is a real experience and an event in
nature, Freud obviously felt more comfortable thinking about it in the
form of nerve impulses. Another example of the difficulties inherent in
Freud's theoretical system is to be found in his thinking about grief
following bereavement. Freud assumed that grief was normal; but he
wondered how to understand the "economics" of grief. In terms of his
theoretical system, "economics" are based on the tendency of the organism to throw off stimulation as quickly as possible. Why, then, *decathecting* a loved person who has died should be so painful was a
puzzle, since decathecting should be pleasurable, not painful. From the
work of modern social anthropologists we now know that grief is universal as well as normal. Human culture universally involves the affectional ties that result in grief at bereavement. We also know that these
same affectional ties breed and are bred by the moral law that is immanent in all human cultures.

Perhaps because he was secularizing guilt and shame, as for example in his analysis of Christoph Haizmann's "demonological neurosis,"
Freud found it difficult to formulate a theory in which emotions would
have equal status in "reality" with electrical charges and physiological
events. Thus Freud described the origin of guilt as the resolution of the
sons' conflict between affection for and hatred of their father. But in his
theory of guilt he was unable to accept his own description of the "primal deed" as a parable, because to do so would involve him in relying
on emotions as prime movers of psychological events. Instead, he insisted on the historical reality of the primal deed, even though that involved
him in a Lamarckian version of hereditary transmission.

Similarly, he abandoned his own clinically accurate description of
the way in which ambivalent feeling is transformed into anxiety, sub-
stituting the theory that anxiety is a cognitive signal of a "real" physical
danger of castration. Once he had made this theoretical commitment,
his view of women's development, which involved no such "real" danger, helped to perpetuate the cultural myth of women's inferiority.

Freud's theoretical system, as set forth in *The Interpretation of
Dreams*, suffered a major blow with the discovery of the REMS. But even

before that happened, Freud's theorizing had become an uncomfortable restraint on research precisely because his theoretical system started with the individual reflex arc instead of with an emotional transaction. When he was describing the work of "primary process" in dreams, Freud likened the censorship to a social-emotional transaction in which one person had to make a "disagreeable remark" to another person on whom the speaker was "dependent." As one result of the contradiction between his observation and his theorizing, primary process is still regarded in some Freudian quarters as "primitive," as contrasted with the higher-order "secondary processes" of "reality testing." This in spite of clear evidence that primary-process transformations in dreams, mistakes, jokes, and neurotic symptoms all involve a high level of intellectual sophistication.

Still, the validity of Freud's descriptions of primary-process transformations of emotional conflict is attested by many cross-cultural validations of the emotional meaning of dream content. Similarly, Freud's descriptions of neurotic symptoms, beginning with hysteria, showed that their content represents not just individual pathology but a powerful critique of the existing social order.

The issue of the nature of human nature has been central in the writings of the psychoanalytic revisionists, beginning with Adler and including Horney, W. Reich, Fromm, and Sullivan, all of whom criticized Freud for his individualistic theory. None of these critics, however, explicitly formulated human nature as social by reason of its cultural nature. Nor have these critics explicitly focused on Freud's descriptions of the power of shame and guilt to create symptoms. Moreover, the concept of "primary narcissism" has recently been revised within the psychoanalytic movement in an effort to reconceptualize difficult cases. As I have already suggested, I think some of these difficult cases of so-called "narcissistic personality" are actually cases in which bypassed shame has not been identified in the patient–therapist relationship and in life. There is a considerable difference between a formulation that conceptualizes cases as narcissistically regressed and one that conceptualizes the consequences of bypassed shame. The latter problem is easier to overcome.

Embedded in the concept of human beings as social creatures is the problem of the distinction between the ego and the self. Each of us is a unique individual; a biologically given system of attachment must ultimately find its way to the individual genetic factors that are the underpinning of each organism, that is, each ego. Yet, since each organism (ego) develops within a social system, it is necessary to recognize the existence of a self that registers and assimilates social interactions. Each unique human self is thus a social product; the self is not to be confused either with "selfishness" or with "narcissism," that is, self-love. Rather, in dialectical fashion, a "secure" and well-differentiated self develops out of an affectional matrix, incorporating a social heritage of affectional bonds into its individualized, independently functioning (social) self.

It is fascinating to consider (see Chapter 6) how close Freud came to having a social theory of human nature, since the examples on which he based his theoretical model of primary process have to do with the infant and its caretaker. But Freud's model started with the "absent" caretaker in the genesis of emotions. In this formulation, positive emotion arises only when it puts an end to internal, instinctive negative emotions. The stimuli to satisfaction are learned through association between them and drive reduction. This is what Bowlby aptly calls the "cupboard-love" theory of human nature: Attachment to the caretaker must be learned through a series of drive-reduction experiences.

Although affects are actually primary motivators in Freud's models, the affects on which the model focuses are the "negative" ones—those that are disorganizing to the smooth functioning of the individual's behavior. This is an emphasis within which one can easily slip, as Freud did, into the hypothesis that *all* affects are inherently disorganizing or "primitive," and that the task of the developing human being is to change affects into "cognitive signals."

A second chain of theorizing is set in motion by a model that starts from the disorganizing negative affects. Because the threatened aggressions in the model imply "real" dangers, the cognitions that accompany the negative affects are understood as valid representations of real-world events, including those arising "within" the organism, as, for instance, hunger. But if the cognitive representations are valid and, by implication, the negative affects "appropriate," how do these veridical cognitions and appropriate affects arise out of disorganization? A tortuous question then arises—one that also plagued Freud: What is the primary force in the development of valid cognition? Negative affect?

Two theoretical models were developed within the Freudian movement to answer this question. In one model, Freud's own (1900, 1926), and in the almost identical model expounded by Anna Freud (1946), all cognitions originate in the negative affect associated with physical danger. By implication, the positive emotions are unknowable.

It was to correct the concept that all cognitions are born out of negative affect that Hartmann offered a second model that included a concept of the "conflict-free" ego-sphere. In a compromise position, Hartmann offered the thesis that some veridical cognitions arise in direct adaptive response to what Hartmann specified as the "average expecta-

ble environment." Had Hartmann's adaptation formula explicitly specified an average expectable *benign social* environment, Freud's description of affects as primary motivators might have been maintained. As it
was formulated, however, Hartmann's correction continued to assume
the individualistic nature of the organism, and a dichotomy between
affect and cognition. It assumed, also, that affect influences cognition
only if it is "negative," and by implication equated affect with "disturbances" of cognition.

Hartmann's correction also left intact that aspect of Freud's theoretical view of the relation between affect and cognition in which the former
is specified as primitive and the latter as an advanced form of human
behavior. Rapaport's effort to systematize psychoanalytic theory by distinguishing between a special clinical theory and a general theory of
human behavior rested on this emphasis in Hartmann. In fact,
Rapaport, following Hartmann, equated primary-process and secondary-process modes of functioning with primitive and more advanced
thinking, respectively. Yet when Freud is describing clinical phenomena, whether symptom, dream content, everyday mistakes, jokes,
or defenses, it is clear that "primary-process" transformations are not
primitive but often very sophisticated ways in which thought symbolizes feeling and vice versa.

It is instructive to speculate (with hindsight) on how Freudian theory might have been formulated had the adaptive exigencies of the nurturant mother and her infant been the guiding principle of evolution.
Smooth emotional bonding would then have become the primary motivation of behavior. Positive and negative affects would be equally
geared to affectional maintenance. Cognition would not be opposed to
affect, but assumed to work coherently with it in order to maintain
bonding. Coherence of affect and cognition is an assumption in both
Tomkins's and Abelson's otherwise differing "script" theories. This coherence of cognition and affect is what Freud actually assumed in his
clinical descriptions of emotional states, but ignored. The vexing problem of which comes first, cognition or affect (Zajonc, 1980), can also be
understood as an artifact resulting from the failure to recognize an attachment system as the framework in which both arise simultaneously.

Another, even more profound reason for the difficulties in Freud's
theoretical system lies in his adherence to Darwinian evolutionary biology (see Chapter 5). Within this framework, partly as a result of androcentric attitudes, there was and still is a heavy emphasis on the adaptive
value of male aggression, that is, skill and cunning in fighting as the
prime selection factor in human evolution. The needs of the nurturant
mother as a factor in the evolution of humanity have tended to be

ignored. This imbalance is only recently being redressed in evolutionary biology, in sociobiology, and in the studies of ethologists. Lovejoy (1981), for example, suggests that humanity's advances in brain development and material culture were the *result*, not the cause, of an "established hominid character system" that included "intensified parenting and social relationships" (p. 348).

Sociobiologists have also attempted to redress this imbalance. For example, they postulate that culture is humanity's major biological adaptation. Anchoring culture in biology, however, can readily become social Darwinism, that is, a doctrine that rationalizes the inequities, oppression, and warfare that characterize many cultures, including our own. Human culture, however, is Janus-faced: It *sometimes* comprises oppression, warfare, and the inferiority of women, but it *always* involves the institutionalized nurturance out of which morality arises. Thus, anchoring morality in biology calls attention to the profoundly social nature of our species, as well as to the destructive capacities that are unleashed when social bonds are threatened. Calling attention to the biology of nurturance can thus be a tool for the critique of the institutionalized oppression and war in particular cultures.

The work of the ethologists calls attention to the social conditions governing even the narrowest neurophysiological responses. Animals' social relationships assume equal if not greater importance than their relationship to their physical surroundings. Close attention to these social conditions has yielded important evidence of a "hedonic" mode of social cohesion among nonhuman primates in which other animals are "positive social referents," in contrast to the "agonic" mode, organized around a dominant male as a response to the threat of danger. Freud shared the prevailing male-centered focus of evolutionary biology. Thus, as we have just seen, his theory of infancy centered on individual responses to an "absent" caretaker rather than on a system of affectional interaction.

A theory of emotions that places them within the human attachment system helps to throw light on a number of problems in both psychoanalysis and mainstream academic psychology. The first of these is the problem of infant competence. Information confirming their competence has increased with remarkable rapidity over the past few years. Infants are much more compentent than suggested either by William James's picture of their "confusion" of by Freud's very similar image of their chaotic id. They are capable of astonishing feats of intellectual response. This relatively new information ceases to be so astonishing when we fit it together with a concept of a "given" infant–caretaker affectional system. Infants are genetically equipped to respond socially, and they are thus capable of much more complex intellectual activities than psychologists had previously imagined.

Neonates, for example, begin to cry when they hear other neonates crying, and neonate girls are a bit more sensitive than boys. Twelve-day-old infants can imitate adult facial expressions. Eighteen to twenty-week old infants can recognize the correspondence between auditorially and visually presented speech sounds; some of them even imitated the sounds presented during one experiment. Infants in the first 7 months of life show facial expressions that signal physical distress as well as the emotions of interest, joy, surprise, sadness, anger, disgust, and fear. These are what Izard has termed the "primary emotions"; they all have signal value for the caretaker, and are universally apprehended in other societies as well as our own.

Infant intellectual, social, and emotional responses are thus enmeshed in the infant–caretaker affectional system. Although the intellectual, social, and emotional descriptions of their behavior may be separately investigated, they are inseparably linked. For example, the intellectual capacity that neonates have to discriminate other neonates' crying from a variety of similar auditory stimuli is indicated by an emotional response, crying, which is also a social response. That neonate girls have something more of this intellectual-social-emotional capacity than do boys indicates the profundity of the social substrate on which human culture is founded and which human culture in turn promotes.

A highly differentiated intellectual-social-emotional life is thus anchored in the infant–caretaker interaction system, as well as in the organism's physiological responses which figured so heavily in James's and Freud's thinking. Attempts to derive attachment, as Freud did, from so-called primary individual instincts or drives have fallen of their own weight, in part because babies are much more organized and socially competent creatures than Freud or the stimulus–response behaviorists, whose theory he was aping, had any way of knowing. As we saw in Chapter 7, observers of the mother–infant interaction who start from a behaviorist learning approach also need an "ethologicosociocognitive" hypothesis it account for "the game" of contingencies and reinforcements out of which infant smiling and cooing evolve. (Again, critics of psychoanalysts for their use of jargon should not exclude behaviorists from similar charges.)

Mothers learn to distinguish in the very early weeks between their infant's so-called "mad" cries and cries resulting from "real" or "just" causes—physical distress or hunger. A process of shaming and guilt induction begins very early with messages about inappropriate protest, about misperceived "rejection." The message that such crying is inappropriate implies that the child is *able* but unwilling to do without mother—in other words, a guilt message. The sequence: rejection → humiliated fury → guilt is thus a normal one, and an adaptive one provided it is experienced in interaction with a stably affectionate and appropriately judging early caretaker, and, later on, in a just world.

A theory of emotions that places them in the framework of an attachment system also helps to ease some problems in the psychology of human development. An uneasy and often unacknowledged consensus exists in modern academia on the proposition that the appropriately affectionate infant–parent interaction is a powerful and pervasive determinant of personality and cognitive style throughout the course of development. Current theorizing suggests, moreover, that the problem of human development is not, as Freud put it, how infant polymorphous primal narcissists (governed by the id) become social creatures, but how narcissists develop out of originally sociable beings. The "secure base" from which the infant develops self-confidence and exploratory behavior is only one example of a robust, fruitful concept derived from Freud's observations, not from his theorizing. Emotional, social, and intellectual development proceed in tandem, anchored in the evolving attachment system, which fosters differentiation and individuation of the self.

A forerunner of the infant–caretaker affectional system is clearly a part of our own primate heritage. As with nonhuman primates, human sexuality is embedded in the matrix of social relationships. Other adult competences are similarly embedded. When Freud made his inspired observation that what we call affection will unfailingly show itself one day in the genitalia (see Chapter 4), he could not know how well his clinical prediction would be borne out by the Harlows' studies, which, like Bowlby's were undertaken in response to his *Three Essays*.

Freud clearly observed that the infant–caretaker interaction is different for the two sexes, if only because girls have a same-sex and boys an opposite-sex caretaker in infancy. Among the most significant and puzzling experimental findings that have developed since Freud raised questions about anatomy and destiny is the sex difference in primate vulnerability to maternal deprivation. Males have been shown to be much more vulnerable to maternal deprivation not only in adult sexual capacity but in a variety of other social behaviors. Although the evidence from our own acculturated species is less unequivocal than that from nonhuman primates, there is more than a suggestion that human male infants are more subject to "inconsolable states" than are females, that mothers have a harder time pacifying their male infants. These experimental findings point to the possibility that some intrinsic, genetic-hormonal difference between the sexes renders females more resistant to

the psychological stress of maternal deprivation. The same line of speculation suggests that women may have a slight edge in the sociability
that is intrinsic in both sexes. It would not be difficult to attribute this
sociability advantage to the genetic-hormonal basis for maternal behavior.

It is interesting to observe, in passing, how androcentric attitudes
still prevail in modern scientific attitudes toward this sex difference.
Maccoby and Jacklin (1974), for example, accept a genetic basis for aggression in males (via the established fact that there is genetic control of
differing hormones in the two sexes). But they do not accord the same
status to the notion that nurturant behavior in women is genetically
based, although they have "no doubt that women throughout the world
are perceived to be the nurturant sex" (p. 215). Their reluctance to accept
the possibility of a genetic base for women's greater sociability may be
understood as stemming not only from the fact that there are fewer
studies of women's sociability than of men's aggression, but from an
understandable fear, which so many feminists share, that information
about women's sociability will be used to "explain" their social inferiority. In any case, the concept of human beings as social by biological
origin, together with the corollary hypothesis that women may be more
social than men, is now a viable theory, as it was not in Freud's time.

A theoretical framework based on the cultural nature of human
nature can accommodate both the genetic sexual differentiation and the
culture's interpretation of women's nurturant function. Such a framework assumes that there will be sex differences in the acculturation
process, based on an interaction between genetics and culturally fostered sex roles—in particular, the scope each culture allows for the sociability of both sexes, and the extent to which the culture assumes the
equality of both sexes. This formulation effects an explicit rapprochement between psychoanalysis and feminism by making use of Freud's
descriptions of primary-process transformations to help unravel the ideology of women's inferiority.

A framework that bases emotions in the attachment system also
helps to make sense out of individual differences in cognitive style,
including sex differences in field dependence and in proneness to shame
and guilt. Freud described personality differences based on the mode of
relatedness of the self to significant others, distinguishing especially
between personality formed around the "external" threat of "loss of
love" and the "internal" threat, "fear of conscience." (Here Freud per-
petuated his hopeless confusion between so-called "external" and "internal" threats.) Field dependence has been used as a tracer element of
differences in the self's modes of relatedness to others and of the self's

relationships to the inanimate or physical world. These are two main tracks of intellectual development as well, and they make different demands upon the organization of the self. In emotional relationships the boundaries between the self and the other are often necessarily fluid; what affects the other person affects the self in empathetic or vicarious experience. In response to the physical or inanimate world, the self's boundaries in relation to things must be sharper and more articulate, that is, more field independent. In cultures where women's activities are confined to childrearing and where women are the servants of men, these two main tracks can become very lopsided in their use.

That stable emotional attachments, formed early, predict a self that is interpersonally adept *and* has well-articulated boundaries is now reasonably well established for young children in our own society. But by adulthood, there is a paradox: Field independence goes not only with cognitive restructuring skills, but with deficits in dealing interpersonally, whereas field dependence goes not only with interpersonal skills but with cognitive restructuring deficits. This is the stereotypical pattern of sex differences, not only in our own society but in many other male-dominated societies as well. The work on field dependence, especially in cross-cultural studies, thus clarifies the way our social order demands different sacrifices from men and women in their relation to the attachment system. As discussed in Volume 1, a different pattern of sacrifice is also visible in women's relative proneness to depression and men's relative proneness to paranoia.

A theory of emotions based on the cultural nature of human nature sees psychiatric symptoms as the means by which people try to remain acculturated in the face of threats to their basic affectional ties. This theoretical framework rests on Freud's *description* of primary-process transformations of shame and guilt into symptoms and into dreams, mistakes, jokes, and defenses. It abandons his *theoretical* account of primary process and his theory of "primary narcissism."

Freud's descriptive focus on the morality immanent in human nature has helped to humanize psychological science. His accurate descriptions of human experience under the stress of the moral emotions of shame and guilt have been one reason for his immeasurable influence on modern psychology and modern thought. To the extent that this book fosters an integration of these descriptions into an adequate theory of human nature it will have accomplished its purpose.

Bibliography

Abelson, R. (1976). Script processing in attitude formation and decision-making. In J. S. Carroll & J. W. Payne (Eds.), *Cognition and social behavior*. Hillsdale, N.J.: Erlbaum.

Abelson, R. (1981). Psychological status of the script concept. *American Psychologist, 36*, 715–730.

Abraham, K. (1924/1965). Character formation on the genital level of development. In *Selected papers of Karl Abraham*. London: Hogarth Press.

Abraham, K. (1927–1965). The influence of oral erotism on character formation. In *Selected Papers of Karl Abraham*. London: Hogarth Press.

Ainsworth, M. (1963). The development of infant–mother interactions among the Ganda. In B. M. Foss (Ed.), *Determinants of infant behavior* (Vol. 2). New York: Wiley.

Ainsworth, M. (1979). Infant–mother attachment. *American Psychologist, 34*, 932–937.

Allport, G. (1943). The ego in contemporary psychology. *Psychological Review, 50*, 451–478.

Asch, S., & Witkin, H. (1948). Studies in space orientation. I, II. *Journal of Experimental Psychology, 38*, 325–337; 455–477.

Aserinsky, E., & Kleitman, N. (1953). Regularly occurring periods of eye motilites, and concomitant phenomena. *Science, 118*, 273–274.

Bakan, D. (1966). *The duality of human existence*. Chicago: Rand McNally.

Bandura, A., & Walters, R. (1959). *Adolescent aggression: A study of the influence of child-training practices and family interrelationships*. New York: Ronald Press.

Barry, H., Child, I., & Bacon, M. (1959). Relations of child training to subsistence economy. *American Anthropologist, 61*, 51–63.

Baumrind, D. (1980). New directions in socialization research. *American Psychologist, 35*, 639–652.

Bayley, N., & Schaefer, E. (1964). Correlations of maternal and child behaviors with the development of mental abilities. *Monographs of the Society for Research in Child Development, 29* (No. 97).

Beach, F. (Ed.) (1965). *Sex and behavior*. New York: Wiley.

Beach, F. (Ed.) (1978). *Human sexuality in four perspectives*. Baltimore, Johns Hopkins Press.

Beck, A. (1967). *Depression: Clinical, experimental and theoretical aspects*. New York: Harper & Row.

Beloff, H. (1957). The structure and origin of the anal character. *Genetic Psychology Monographs, 55*, 141–172.

217

Bem, S. (1975). Sex-role adaptability: One consequence of psychological androgyny. *Journal of Personality and Social Psychology, 31,* 634–643.

Bem, S. (1976). Probing the promise of androgyny. In A. Kaplan, & J. Bean, (Eds.), *Beyond sex-role stereotypes: Probing the promise of androgyny.* Boston: Little, Brown.

Bem, S., Martyna, W., & Watson, C. (1976). Sex typing and androgyny: Further explorations of the expressive domain. *Journal of Personality and Social Psychology, 34,* 1016–1023.

Benedict, R. (1946). *The chrysanthemum and the sword.* New York: Houghton Mifflin.

Berger, R. (1963). Experimental modifications of dream content by meaningful verbal stimuli. *British Journal of Psychiatry, 109,* 722–740.

Berger, R. (1967). *Eye movements during paradoxical sleep following different conditional roles of eye movements during watchfulness in Macaca nemestoma.* Paper presented at the Meeting of the Association for the Psychophysiological Study of Sleep, Santa Monica.

Berger, R., & Oswald, I. (1962). Eye movements during active and passive dreams. *Science, 136,* 601.

Bernstein, I. (1978). Sex differences in the behaviors of non-human primates. *Social Science and Medicine, 12,* 151–155.

Berry, J. (1976). *Human ecology and cognitive style.* New York: Wiley.

Bertini, M., Lewis, H., & Witkin, H. (1964). [Some preliminary observations with an experimental procedure for the study of hypnagogic and related phenomena.] *Archivio di Psychologica, Neurologica e Psychiatrica, 6,* 493–534.

Blasi, A. (1980). Bridging moral cognition and moral action. A critical review of the literature. *Psychological Bulletin, 88,* 1–45.

Blum, G. (1963). *Psychoanalytic theories of personality.* New York: McGraw-Hill.

Bokert, E. G. (1968). The effects of thirst and a related verbal stimulus on dream reports. *Dissertation Abstracts,* 4753B.

Bone, R., Thomas, T., & Kinsolving, D. (1972). Relationship of rod and frame scores to dream recall. *Psychological Reports, 30,* 58.

Bourdieu, P. (1966). The sentiment of honor in Kabyle society. In J. Peristiany (Ed.), *Honour and shame: Values of a Mediterranean society.* Chicago: University of Chicago Press.

Bowlby, J. (1969, 1980). *Attachment and loss* (Vol. 1,3). *New York:* Basic Books.

Brenman, M., & Gill, M. (1947). *Hypnotherapy.* New York: Wiley.

Breuer, J., & Freud, S. (1893–1895). Studies on hysteria. In J. Strachey (Ed.), *Standard edition: The complete psychological works of Sigmund Freud* (Vol. 2). London: Hogarth Press.

Broughton, R. (1968). Sleep disorders: Disorders of arousal? *Science, 159,* 1070–1078.

Brownmiller, S. (1975). *Against our will: Men, women and rape.* New York: Simon & Schuster.

Burton, R., & Whiting, J. (1961). The absent father and cross-sex identity. *Merrill-Palmer Quarterly, 7,* 85–95.

Byrne, D. (1964). Repression–sensitization and dimensions of personality. *Progress in Experimental Psychology, 1,* 169–220.

Cartwright, R., & Monroe, L. (1967). *The relation of dreaming and REM-sleep: The effects of REM deprivation under two conditions.* Paper presented at the meeting of the Association for the Psychophysiological Study of Sleep, Santa Monica.

Cartwright, R., Monroe, L., & Palmer, C. (1967). Individual differences in response to REM-deprivation. *Archives of General Psychiatry, 16,* 297–303.

Castaldo, V., & Holzman, R. (1967). The effects of hearing one's own voice on sleep mentation. *Journal of Nervous and Mental Disease, 144,* 2–13.

Chance, M. (1980). An ethological assessment of emotion. In R. Plutchik & H. Kellerman (Eds.), *Emotion: Theory, research and experience.* New York: Academic Press.

Chassaguet-Smirgel, J. (1970). *Female sexuality.* Ann Arbor: University of Michigan Press.

Chein, I. (1944). Awareness of the self and the structure of the ego. *Psychological Review, 51,* 304–314.

Chodorow, N. (1971). Being and doing: A cross-cultural examination of the socialization of males and females. In V. Gornick & B. Moran (Eds.), *Woman in sexist society.* New York: New American Library.

Chodorow, N. (1978). *The reproduction of mothering.* Berkeley: University of California Press.

Cohen, Y. (1978). The disappearance of the incest taboo. *Human Nature, 1,* 72–78.

Constantinople, A. (1973). Masculinity-femininity: An exception to a famous dictum. *Psychological Bulletin, 80,* 389–407.

D'Andrade, R. G. (1961). The effect of culture on dreams. In F. Hsu (Ed.), *Psychological anthropology: Approaches to culture and personality.* Dorsey Press.

Darwin, C. (1871). *The descent of man and selection in relation to sex.* London: Murray.

Daube, D. (1969). The culture of deuteronomy. *Orita, 3,* 27–52.

Davenport, W. (1978). Sex in cross-cultural perspective. In F. Beach (Ed.), *Human sexuality in four perspectives.* Baltimore: Johns Hopkins Press.

De Casper, A., & Fifer, W. (1980). Of human bonding: Newborns prefer their mothers' voices. *Science, 208,* 1174–1176.

Dement, W. (1955). Dream recall and eye movements during sleep in schizophrenics and normals. *Journal of Nervous and Mental Disease, 122,* 263–269.

Dement, W. (1966). The psychophysiology of sleep and dreams. In S. Arieti (Ed.), *American handbook of psychiatry* (Vol. 3). New York: Basic Books.

Dement, W. (1969). The biological role of REM sleep (circa 1968). In A. Kales (Ed.), *Sleep: Physiology and pathology.* Philadelphia: Lippincott

Dement, W., & Wolpert, J. (1958). The relation of eye movements, bodily mobility and external structure to dream content. *Journal of Experimental Psychology, 55,* 543–553.

Dinnerstein, D. (1977). *The mermaid and the minotaur.* New York: Harper & Row.

Dodds, E. (1951). *The Greeks and the irrational.* Oxford: Oxford University Press.

Dollard, J., Doob, L., Miller, N., Mowrer, O., & Sears, R. (1939). *Frustration and aggression.* New Haven: Yale University Press.

Domhoff, B., & Kamiya, J. (1964). Problems in dream content study with objective indicators. *Archives of General Psychiatry, 11,* 525–532.

DuBois, C. (1944). *The people of Alor.* Minneapolis: University of Minnesota Press.

Edel, A. (1980). *Exploring fact and value* (Vol. 2). New Brunswick, N.J.: Transaction Books.

Edel, L. (1964). *The modern psychological novel* (Rev. ed.). New York: Grosset & Dunlap.

Edel, M., & Edel, A. (1968). *Anthropology and ethics* (Rev. ed.). Cleveland: Western Reserve Press.

Engels, F. (1884). *The origin of the family, private property and the state.* New York: International Publishers.

Ephron, H., & Carrington, P. (1966). Rapid eye movement sleep and cortical homeostasis. *Psychological Review, 73,* 500–526.

Erdelyi, M. (1974). A new look at the new look: Perceptual defense and vigilance. *Psychological Review, 81,* 1–26.

Eriksen, C. W. (1963). Perception and personality. In J. M. Wepman & K. W. Heine (Eds.), *Concepts of personality.* Chicago: Aldine.

Erikson, E. (1950). *Childhood and society.* New York: W. W. Norton.

Erikson, E. (1954). The dream specimen of psychoanalysis. *Journal of the American Psychological Association, 2,* 5–59.

Erikson, E. (1964). Inner and outer space: Reflections on womanhood. *Daedalus, 93,* 582–606.

Federn, P. (1952). *Ego psychology and the psychoses.* New York: Basic Books.

Feinberg, I. (1968). Eye movement activity during sleep and intellectual function on mental retardation. *Science, 159,* 1256.

Feinberg, I., Koresko, R., & Gottlieb, F. (1965). Further observations on electrophysiological sleep patterns in schizophrenia. *Comprehensive Psychiatry, 6,* 21–24.

Fenichel, O. (1945). *The psychoanalytic theory of neuroses.* New York: W. W. Norton.

Field, T., Woodson, R., Greenberg, R., & Cohen, D. (1982). Discrimination and imitation of facial expression by neonates. *Science, 218,* 179–181.

Finney, J. (1963). Maternal influences on anal or oral character in children. *Journal of Genetic Psychology, 103,* 351–367.

Fisher, C. (1956). A study of the preliminary stages of construction of dreams and images. *Journal of the American Psychoanalytic Association, 4,* 5–48.

Fisher, C., Schiavi, R., Lear, H., Edwards, A., Davis, D., & Witkin, A. (1975). The assessment of nocturnal REM erection in the differential diagnosis of sexual impotence. *Journal of Sex and Marital Therapy, 1.*

Fisher, S., & Greenberg, R. (1977). *The scientific credibility of Freud's theories and therapy.* New York: Basic Books.

Fliegel, Z. (1973. Feminine psychosexual development in Freudian theory: A historical reconstruction. *Psychoanalytic Quarterly, 42,* 385–408.

Fliegel, Z. (1982). Half a century later: Current status of Freud's controversial views on women. *Psychoanalytic Review, 69,* 7–28.

Ford, C., & Beach, F. (1951). *Patterns of sexual behavior.* New York: Harper.

Foulkes, D., Pivik, T., Ahrens, J., and Swanson, E. (1968). Effects of "dream-deprivation" on dream content: An attempted cross-night replication. *Journal of Abnormal Psychology, 73,* 403–415.

Foulkes, W., & Rechtschaffen, A. (1964). Pre-sleep determinants of dream content: Effects of two films. *Perceptual and Motor Skills, 19,* 983–1005.

Freud, A. (1946). *The ego and mechanisms of defence.* New York: International Universities Press.

Freud, S. (1894). The neuro-psychoses of defence. In J. Strachey (Ed.), *Standard edition* (Vol. 3). London: Hogarth Press.

Freud, S. (1896). Further remarks on the neuro-psychoses of defence. In J. Strachey (Ed.), *Standard edition* (Vol. 3). London: Hogarth Press.

Freud, S. (1899). Screen memories. In J. Strachey (Ed.), *Standard Edition* (Vol. 3). London: Hogarth Press.

Freud, S. (1900). The interpretation of dreams. In J. Strachey (Ed.), *Standard edition* (Vol. 5). London: Hogarth Press.

Freud, S. (1901a). On dreams. In J. Strachey (Ed.), *Standard edition* (Vol. 5). London: Hogarth Press.

Freud, S. (1901b). The psychopathology of everyday life. In J. Strachey (Ed.), *Standard edition* (Vol. 6). London: Hogarth Press

Freud, S. (1905a). Jokes and their relation to the unconscious. In J. Strachey (Ed.), *Standard edition* (Vol. 8). London: Hogarth Press

Freud, S. (1905b). Three essays on the theory of sexuality. In J. Strachey (Ed.), *Standard edition* (Vol. 7). London: Hogarth Press

Freud, S. (1908a). Character and anal-erotism. In J. Strachey (Ed.), *Standard edition* (Vol. 9). London: Hogarth Press.

Freud, S. (1908b). Civilized sexual morality and modern nervous illness. In J. Strachey (Ed.), *Standard edition* (Vol. 9). London: Hogarth Press.

Freud, S. (1909). Notes upon a case of obsessional neurosis. In J. Strachey (Ed.), *Standard edition* (Vol. 10). London: Hogarth Press.

Freud, S. (1910). Five lectures on psychoanalysis. In J. Strachey (Ed.), *Standard edition* (Vol. 11). London: Hogarth Press.

Freud, S. (1913). Totem and taboo. In J. Strachey (Ed.), *Standard edition* (Vol. 13). London: Hogarth Press.

Freud, S. (1914). On narcissism: An introduction. In J. Strachey (Ed.), *Standard edition* (Vol. 14). London: Hogarth Press.

Freud, S. (1915a) Instincts and their vicissitudes. In J. Strachey (Ed.), *Standard edition* (Vol. 14). London: Hogarth Press.

Freud, S. (1915b). Repression. In J. Strachey (Ed.), *Standard edition* (Vol. 14). London: Hogarth Press.

Freud, S. (1915c). Thoughts on war and death. In J. Strachey (Ed.), *Standard edition* (Vol. 14). London: Hogarth Press.

Freud, S. (1915–1916). Introductory lectures on psychoanalysis. In J. Strachey (Ed.), *Standard edition* (Vol. 15). London: Hogarth Press.

Freud, S. (1916). Some character-types met with in psychoanalytic work. In J. Strachey (Ed.), *Standard edition* (Vol. 14). London: Hogarth Press.

Freud, S. (1918). The taboo of virginity. In J. Strachey (Ed.), *Standard edition* (Vol. 11). London: Hogarth Press.

Freud, S. (1920). Beyond the pleasure principle. In J. Strachey (Ed.), *Standard edition* (Vol. 18). London: Hogarth Press.

Freud, S. (1921). Group psychology and the analysis of the ego. In J. Strachey (Ed.), *Standard edition* (Vol. 18). London: Hogarth Press.

Freud, S. (1925). Some psychical consequences of the anatomical distinction between the sexes. In J. Strachey (Ed.), *Standard edition* (Vol. 19). London: Hogarth Press.

Freud, S. (1926). Inhibitions, symptoms and anxiety. In J. Strachey (Ed.), *Standard edition* (Vol. 20). London: Hogarth Press.

Freud, S. (1927a). The future of an illusion. In J. Strachey (Ed.), *Standard edition* (Vol. 21). London: Hogarth Press.

Freud, S. (1927b). Humour. In J. Strachey (Ed.), *Standard edition* (Vol. 21). London: Hogarth Press.

Freud, S. (1930). Civilization and its discontents. In J. Strachey (Ed.), *Standard edition* (Vol. 21). London: Hogarth Press.

Freud, S. (1931). On libidinal types. In J. Strachey (Ed.), *Standard edition* (Vol. 21). London: Hogarth Press.

Freud, S. (1933). New introductory lectures on psychoanalysis. In J. Strachey (Ed.), *Standard edition* (Vol. 22). London: Hogarth Press.

Freud, S., & Oppenheim, E. (1911). In J. Strachey (Ed.), *Standard edition* (Vol. 12). London: Hogarth Press.

Fromm, E. (1941). *Escape from freedom.* New York: Farrar & Rinehart.

Fromm, E. (1943). Sex and character. *Psychiatry, 6,* 21–31.

Fromm, E. (1955). *The sane society.* New York: Rinehart.

Gibson, J., & Mowrer, D. (1938). Determinants of the perceived vertical and horizontal. *Psychological Review, 45,* 300–323.

Gilligan, C. (1981). *In a different voice.* Cambridge: Harvard University Press, 1981.

Gilligan, C. (1983). Do the social sciences have an adequate theory of moral development? In N. Haan, R. Bellah, P. Rabinow, & W. Sullivan (Eds.), *Social science as moral inquiry.* New York: Columbia University Press.

Gleser, G., & Ihilevich, D. (1969). An objective instrument for measuring defense mechanisms. *Journal of Consulting and Clinical Psychology, 33,* 51–60.

Glover, E. (1956). *On the early development of mind.* New York: International Universities Press.

Goldman-Eisler, F. (1948). Breast-feeding and character formation. *Journal of Personality, 17,* 83–103.

Goldman-Eisler, F. (1950). Breast-feeding and character formation. *Journal of Personality, 19,* 189–196.

Goldman-Eisler, F. (1951). The problem of "orality" and its origin in early childhood. *Journal of Mental Science, 97,* 765–782.

Goodenough, D. (1967). Some recent studies of dream recall. In H. Witkin & H. Lewis, (Eds.), *Experimental studies of dreaming.* New York: Random House.

Goodenough, D., Lewis, H., Shapiro, A., Jaret, L., & Sleser, I. (1965). Dream reporting following abrupt and gradual awakenings from different types of sleep. *Journal of Personality and Social Psychology, 2,* 170–179.

Goodenough, D., Witkin, H., Lewis, H., Koulack, D., & Cohen, H. (1974). Repression, interference and field dependence as factors in dream forgetting. *Journal of Abnormal Psychology, 83,* 32–44.

Gottschalk, L., & Gleser, G. (1969). *The measurement of psychological states through the content analysis of verbal behavior.* Berkeley: University of California Press.

Haan, N. (1978). Two moralities in action contexts: Relationships to thought, ego regulation and development. *Journal of Personality and Social Psychology, 36,* 286–306.

Haeberle, E. (1978). Children, sex and society. *Hustler,* December.

Hall, C., & Domhoff, B. (1964). Friendliness in dreams. *Journal of Social Psychology, 62,* 309–314.

Hall, C., & VandeCastle, R. (1966). *The content analysis of dreams.* New York: Appleton-Century-Crofts.

Harlow, H., & Mears, C. (1979). *The human model: Primate perspectives.* New York: Wiley.

Hartmann, E. (1969). Mania, depression and sleep. In A. Kales (Ed.), *Sleep: Psychology and pathology.* Philadelphia: Lippincott.

Hartmann, H. (1951). Ego psychology and the problem of adaptation. In D. Rapaport (Ed.), *Organization and pathology of thought.* New York: Columbia University Press.

Hauri, P., & VandeCastle, R. (1970). *Dream content and physiological arousal during REMS.* Paper presented at the meeting of the Association for the Psychophysiological Study of Sleep, Santa Monica.

Heinstein, M. (1963). Behavioral correlates of breast-bottle regimes under varying parent-infant relationships. *Monographs of the Society for Research in Child Development, 28,* No. 88.

Herman, J. (1981). *Father-daughter incest.* Cambridge: Harvard University Press.

Hersch, R., Antrobus, J., Arkin, A., & Singer, J. L. (1970). Daydreaming as a sympathetic arousal. *Psychophysiology, 7,* 329.

Hoffman, M. (1977). Moral internalization: Current theory and research. In L. Berkowitz (Ed.), *Advances in experimental social psychology* (Vol. 10). New York: Academic Press.

Hogan, R. (1975). Theoretical egocentrism and the problem of compliance. *American Psychologist, 27,* 533–540.

Horney, K. (1932) [1967]. The dread of women. In H. Kelman (Ed.), *Feminine psychology*. New York: W. W. Norton.

Horney, K. (1926 [1967]). The flight from womanhood. In H. Kelman (Ed.), *Feminine psychology*. New York: W. W. Norton.

Horney, K. (1922 [1967]). On the genesis of the castration complex in women. In H. Kelman (Ed.), *Feminine psychology*. New York: W. W. Norton.

Jahoda, M. (1977). *Freud and the dilemmas of psychology*. New York: Basic Books.

Jenkins, C., Rosenman, R., & Friedman, M. (1967). Development of an objective psychological test for the determination of coronary-prone behavior pattern in employed men. *Journal of Chronic Disease, 20*, 371–379.

Jenkins, C., Zyzanski, S., Ryan, T., Flessas, A., & Tannenbaum, S. (1977). Social insecurity and coronary-prone Type A response as identifiers of severe atherosclerosis. *Journal of Consulting and Clinical Psychology 45*, 1060–1067.

Jones, E. (1950). Freud's theory of dreams. In *Papers on psychoanalysis* (5th ed.). London: Balliere, Tandall & Cox. (Revised from *American Journal of Psychology*, 1910, 21).

Jones, E. (1954). *The life and works of Sigmund Freud*. New York: Basic Books.

Jones, E. (1924). Mother-right and the ignorance of savages. In *Essays in applied psychoanalysis*. New York: International Universities Press.

Jones, R. (1974). *The new psychology of dreaming*. New York: Viking Press.

Kagan, J., & Moss, H. (1962). *Birth to maturity: A study in psychological development*. New York: Wiley.

Karacen, I., Goodenough, D., Shapiro, A., & Starker, S. (1966). Erection cycle during sleep in relation to dream anxiety. *Archives of General Psychiatry, 15*, 183–189.

Kardiner, A. (1939). *The individual and his society*. New York: Columbia University Press.

Kinsey, A., Pomeroy, W., & Martin, C. (1948). *Sexual behavior in the human male*. Philadelphia: W. B. Saunders.

Kinsey, A., Pomeroy, W., Martin, C., & Gebhard, P. (1953). *Sexual behavior in the human female*. Philadelphia: W. B. Saunders.

Klein, M. (1948). *Contributions to psychoanalysis, 1921–1945*. London: Hogarth.

Kline, P. (1971). *Fact and fantasy in Freudian theory*. London: Methuen.

Kogan, N. (1976). *Cognitive styles in infancy and early childhood*. New York: Wiley.

Kohlberg, L. (1966). A cognitive-developmental analysis of children's sex-role concepts and attitudes. In E. Maccoby (Ed.), *The development of sex differences*. Stanford, Calif.: Stanford University Press.

Korner, T. (1969). Neonatal startles, smiles, erections and reflex sucks as related to state, sex and individuality. *Child Development, 40*, 1039–1058.

Kramer, M., Whitman, R., Baldridge, W., & Lansky, L. (1966). Dreaming in the depressed. *Canadian Psychiatric Association Journal, 2*, 178–192.

Kramer, M., Whitman, R., & Winget, C. (1970). A survey approach to normative dream content: Sex, age, marital status, race and educational differences. *Psychophysiology, 7*, 325.

Kris, E. (1952). *Psychoanalytic explorations in art*. New York: International Universities Press.

Kubie, L. (1943). The use of induced hypnagogic reveries in the recovery of repressed amnesic data. *Bulletin of the Menninger Clinic, 1*, 172–182.

Kubie, L., & Margolin, S. (1942). A physiological method for the induction of states of partial sleep and securing free associations and early memories in such states. *Transactions of the American Neurological Association*, 136–139.

Lacan, J. (1975). *The language of the self*. New York: Delta Books.

LaFrance, M., & Carmen, B. (1980). The non-verbal display of psychological androgyny. *Journal of Personality and Social Psychology, 38*, 36–49.

Langer, E., & Abelson, R. (1972). The semantics of asking a favor: How to succeed in getting help without really dying. *Journal of Personality and Social Psychology, 24,* 26–32.

Langs, R. (1965). Earliest memories and personality: A predictive study. *Archives of General Psychiatry, 12,* 379–390.

Langs, R. (1966). Manifest dreams from three clinical groups. *Archives of General Psychiatry, 14,* 634–643.

Lazarus, R., Speisman, J., Mordkoff, A., & Davison, L. (1962). A laboratory study of psychological stress produced by a motion picture film. *Psychological Monographs, 76,* No. 533.

Lerner, B. (1966). Rorschach movement and dreams: A validation study using drug-induced dream deprivation. *Journal of Abnormal Psychology, 71,* 75–86.

Lerner, B. (1967). Dream function reconsidered. *Journal of Abnormal Psychology, 72,* 85–100.

Levine, J. (1979). Humor and psychopathology. In C. Izard & J. Singer (Eds.), *Emotions in personality and psychopathology.* New York: Plenum Press.

Lévi-Strauss, C. (1949). *The elementary structures of kinship.* Boston: Beacon Press.

Lévi-Strauss, C. (1967). *Structural anthropology.* New York: Doubleday.

Lévi-Strauss, C. (1968). *The savage mind.* Chicago: University of Chicago Press.

Lévi-Strauss, C. (1962 [1969]). *Totemism.* Middlesex, U.K.: Pelican Books.

Lewis, H. B. (1959). Organization of the self as reflected in manifest dreams. *Psychoanalysis and the Psychoanalytic Review, 46,* 21–35.

Lewis, H. B. (1970). The royal road to the unconscious: Changing conceptualizations of the dream. *International Psychiatry Clinics, 7,* 199–213.

Lewis, H. B. (1971). *Shame and guilt in neurosis.* New York: International Universities Press.

Lewis, H. B., Goodenough, D., Shapiro, A., & Sleser, I. (1966). Individual differences in dream recall. *Journal of Abnormal Psychology, 71,* 52–59.

Lewis, H. B. (1958). Over-differentiation and under-individuation of the self. *Psychoanalysis and the Psychoanalytic Review, 45,* 3–24.

Lewis, H. B. (1976). *Psychic war in men and women.* New York: New York University Press.

Lewis, H. B. (1980). "Narcissistic personality" or "shame-prone" superego modes. *Comprehensive Psychotherapy, 1,* 59–80.

Lewis, H. B. (1981). Shame and guilt in human nature. In S. Tuttman, C. Kaye, & M. Zimmerman (Eds.), *Object and self: A developmental approach. Essays in honor of Edith Jacobson.* New York: International Universities Press.

Lewis, H. B., Goodenough, D., Shapiro, A., & Sleser, I. (1966). Individual differences in dream recall. *Journal of Abnormal Psychology, 71,* 52–54.

Lewis, M., & Brooks-Gunn, J. (1979). *Social cognition and the acquisition of self.* New York: Plenum Press.

Loevinger, J. (1976). *Ego development: Conceptions and theories.* California: Jossey-Bass.

Lovejoy, O. (1981). The origin of man. *Science, 216,* 341.

Lynd, H. (1958). *On shame and the search for identity.* New York: Harcourt, Brace.

Lynn, D. (1961). Sex role and parental identification. *Child Development, 33,* 555–564.

Maccoby, E., & Jacklin, C. (1974). *The psychology of sex differences.* Stanford, Calif.: Stanford University Press.

Madison, P. (1961). *Freud's concept of repression and defence.* Minneapolis: University of Minnesota Press.

Malinowski, B. (1927). *Sex and repression in savage society.* London: Routledge & Kegan Paul.

Martin, K., & Voorhies, B. (1975). *Female of the species.* New York: Columbia University Press.

Masters, W., & Johnson, V. (1970). *Human sexual inadequacy.* Boston: Little, Brown.

Mayman, M. (1968). Early memories and character structure. *Journal of Projective Techniques and Personality Assessment, 32,* 303–316.

Mead, M. (1949). *Male and female.* New York: Morrow.

Minard, J. (1965). Response-bias interpretation of "perceptual defense." *Psychological Review, 72,* 74–88.

Mischel, W. (1966). A social-learning view of the differences in behavior. In E. Maccoby (Ed.), *The development of sex differences.* Stanford, Calif.: Stanford University Press.

Mitchell, J. (1974). *Psychoanalysis and feminism.* New York: Pantheon Books.

Money, J. (Ed.). (1965). *Sex research: New developments.* New York: Holt, Rinehart & Winston.

Morgan, E. (1973). *The descent of woman.* New York: Bantam Books.

Moss, H. (1974). Early sex differences and the mother-infant interaction. In R. Friedman, R. Reichert, & R. Vandeweile (Eds.), *Sex differences in behavior.* New York: Wiley.

Novikoff, A. (1945). The concept of integrative levels and biology. *Science, 101,* 209–215.

Parsons, A. (1964). Is the oedipus complex universal? *Psychoanalytic Study of Society, 3,* 278–328.

Parsons, T. (1958). Social structure and the development of personality: Freud's contribution to the integration of psychology and sociology. *Psychiatry, 21,* 321–340.

Parsons, T. (1964). *Social structure and personality.* Glencoe, Ill.: Free Press.

Piaget, J. (1932). *The moral judgment of the child.* Glencoe, Ill.: Free Press.

Piers, G., & Singer, M. (1953). *Shame and guilt.* Springfield, Ill.: Charles C Thomas.

Pivik, T., & Foulkes, D. (1966). "Dream deprivation": Effects on dream content. *Science, 153,* 1282–1284.

Pomeroy, W. (1976). Incest: A new look. *Forum,* December.

Poetzl, O., Allers, R., & Teler, J. (1960). Preconscious stimulation in dreams, associations and images. In *Psychological Issues Monograph Series* (Vol. 2, No. 3). New York: International Universities Press.

Puner, H. (1978 [1947]). *Freud: His life and times.* New York: Charter Books.

Rapaport, D. (Ed.). (1951). *Organization and pathology of thought.* New York: Columbia University Press.

Rapaport, D. (1960). The structure of psychoanalytic theory. In *Psychological Issues Monograph Series* (Vol. 2, No. 6). New York: International Universities Press.

Rapaport, D. (1968). The psychoanalytic theory of emotions. In M. Arnold (Ed.), *The nature of emotion.* London: Penguin Books.

Reich, W. (1971). *The mass psychology of fascism.* New York: Farrar, Straus & Giroux.

Rheingold, H. (1969). the social and socializing infant. In D. Goslin (Ed.), *Handbook of socialization theory and research.* Chicago: Rand, McNally & Co.

Richardson, G., & Moore, R. (1963). On the manifest dream in schizophrenia. *Journal of the American Psychoanalytic Association, 11,* 281–303.

Robbins, P., & Tanck, R. (1970). The repression-sensitization scale, dreams and dream associations. *Journal of Clinical Psychology, 26,* 219–221.

Roffwarg, H., Muzio, J., & Dement, W. (1966). Ontogenetic development of the human sleep-dream. *Science, 152,* 604–619.

Roheim, G. (1945). *The external ones of the dream.* New York: International Universities Press.

Rorschach, H. (1946 [1921]). *Psychodiagnostics.* New York: Grune & Stratton.

Rosenzweig, S. (1938). The experimental study of repression. In H. A. Murray (Ed.), *Explorations in personality.* New York: Oxford University Press.

Rotter, J. (1966). Generalized expectancies in internal and external control of reinforcement. *Psychological Monographs, 80,* No. 609.

Rousseau, J. (1964). Essay on the origin and foundation of inequality among men. In R. Masters (Ed.), *The first and second discourses*. New York: St. Martin's Press.

Rubin, G. (1975). The traffic in women: Notes on the "political economy of sex." In R. Reiter (Ed.), *Toward an anthropology of women*. New York: Monthly Review Press.

Rubin, J., Provenzano, F., & Luria, Z. (1974). The eye of the beholder: Parents' views on sex of newborns. *American Journal of Orthopsychiatry, 44*, 512–519.

Rutter, M. (1972). *Maternal deprivation reassessed*. London: Penguin Books.

Sackett, G. (1974). Sex differences in rhesus monkeys following varied rearing experiences. In R. Friedman, R. Reichert, & R. Vandeweile (Eds.), *Sex differences in behavior*. New York: Wiley.

Sampson, H. (1965). Deprivation of dreaming sleep by two methods: Compensatory REM-time. *Archives of General Psychiatry, 13*, 79–86.

Sandler, J., & Hazari, A. (1960). The obsessional: On the psychological classification of obsessional character traits and symptoms. *British Journal of Medical Psychology, 33*, 113–121.

Schafer, R. (1954). *Psychoanalytic interpretation in Rorschach testing*. New York: Grune & Stratton.

Schafer, R. (1960). The loving and beloved superego in Freud's structural theory. *Psychoanalytic Study of the Child, 15*, 163–188.

Schimek, J. (1968). Cognitive styles and defences: A longitudinal study of intellectualizations and field independence. *Journal of Abnormal Psychology, 73*, 575–580.

Schonbar, R. (1965). Differential dream recall frequency as a component of "life style." *Journal of Consulting Psychology, 29*, 468–474.

Schroetter, K. (1951). In D. Rapaport (Ed.), *Organization and pathology of thought*. New York: Columbia University Press.

Sears, R., Rau, L., & Alpert, R. (1965). *Identification and child-rearing*. Stanford, Calif.: Stanford University Press.

Seay, B., Hansen, E., & Harlow, H. (1962). Mother-infant separation in monkeys. *Journal of Child Psychology and Psychiatry, 3*, 123–132.

Shapiro, A., Goodenough, D., Lewis, H., & Sleser, I. (1965). Gradual arousal from sleep: A determinant of thinking reports. *Psychosomatic Medicine, 27*, 342–349.

Sharpe, E. (1949). *Dream analysis*. London: Hogarth Press.

Sherfey, M. (1972). *The nature and evolution of female sexuality*. New York: Random House.

Shevrin, H., & Luborsky, L. (1958). The measurement of preconscious perception in dreams and images: An investigation of the Poetzl phenomenon. *Journal of Abnormal and Social Psychology, 56*, 285–294.

Silberer, H. (1951 [1912]). Report on a method of eliciting and observing certain symbolic hallucination-phenomena. In D. Rapaport (Ed.), *Organization and pathology of thought*. New York: Columbia University Press.

Singer, J., & Schonbar, R. (1961). Correlates of day-dreaming: A dimension of self-awareness. *Journal of Consulting Psychology, 25*, 1–7.

Slater, P., & Slater, D. (1965). Maternal ambivalence and narcissism. *Merrill-Palmer Quarterly, 11*, 241–259.

Snyder, F. (1966). Toward an evolutionary theory of dreaming. *American Journal of Psychiatry, 123*, 121–142.

Snyder, F. (1967). In quest of dreaming. In H. Witkin & H. Lewis (Eds.), *Experimental studies of dreaming*. New York: Random House.

Snyder, F., Karacen, I., Tharp, V., & Scott, J. (1967). *Phenomenology of REM dreaming*. Paper presented at the meeting of the Association for the Psychophysiological Study of Sleep, Santa Monica.

Spitz, R. (1945). Hospitalism: An inquiry into the causes of psychoanalytic conditions in early childhood. *Psychoanalytic Study of the Child, 1*, 53–74.

Spitz, R., & Wolf, K. (1946). Anaclitic depression: An inquiry into the causes of psychiatric conditions in early childhood. *Psychoanalytic Study of the Child, 2*, 313–342.

Spitz, R., & Wolf, K. (1949). Autoerotism: Some empirical findings and hypotheses on three of the manifestations in the first year of life. *Psychoanalytic Study of the Child, 3–4*.

Stern, J., Caldwell, B., Hersher, L., Lipton, E., & Richmond, J. (1969). A factor analytic study of the mother–infant dyad. *Child Development, 40*, 161–181.

Stoller, R. (1968). *Sex and gender*. New York: Jason Aronson.

Stoller, R. (1975). *Perversion: The erotic form of hatred*. New York: Pantheon Books.

Stone, L., Smith, H., and Murphy, L. (1978). *The social infant*. New York: Basic Books.

Storms, M. (1980). Theories of sexual orientation. *Journal of Personality and Social Psychology, 38*, 783–793.

Tart, C. (1962). Frequency of dream recall and some personality measures. *Journal of Consulting Psychology, 26*, 467–470.

Tawney, R. H. (1926). *Religion and the rise of capitalism*. New York: Harcourt, Brace.

Tobach, E., & Rosoff, B. (Eds.). (1978). *Genes and gender*. New York: Gordian Press.

Tomkins, S. (1980). Script theory: Differential magnifications of affects. In H. E. Howe, Jr., & M. M. Page (Eds.), *Nebraska Symposium on Motivation* (Vol. 27). Lincoln: University of Nebraska Press.

Turiel, E. (1967). An historical analysis of the Freudian concept of the superego. *Psychoanalytic Review, 54*, 118–140.

Waldron, I. (1978). Type A behavior pattern and coronary heart disease in men and women. *Social Science and Medicine, 12B*, 167–170.

Watson, G. (1973). Smiling, cooing and "the game." *Merrill-Palmer Quarterly, 18*, 323–339. (Reprinted in L. Stone, H. Smith, and L. Murphy (Eds.), *The social infant*. New York: Basic Books.

Weber, M. (1958). *From Max Weber: Essays on sociology* (H. Gerth & C. Mills, Eds.). New York: Oxford University Press.

Weisz, R., & Foulkes, D. (1970). Home and laboratory dreams collected under uniform sampling conditions. *Psychophysiology, 6*, 588–596.

White, R. W. (1959). Motivation reconsidered: The concepts of competence. *Psychological Review, 66*, 297–333.

Whiting, J., & Child, I. (1953). *Child training and personality*. New Haven: Yale University Press.

Wilson, A. & Fromm, E. (In press). Children of holocaust survivors.

Witkin, H. (1965). Psychological differentiation and forms of pathology. *Journal of Abnormal Psychology, 70*, 317–336.

Witkin, H. (1970). Individual differences in dreaming. *International Psychiatric Clinic, 7*, 154, 164.

Witkin, H., & Asch, S. (1948). Studies on space orientation. III and IV. *Journal of Experimental Psychology, 38*, 603–614; 762–782.

Witkin, H., & Berry, J. (1975). Psychological differentiation in cross-cultural perspective. *Journal of Cross-Cultural Psychology, 6*, 4–87.

Witkin, H., & Lewis, H. (1965). The relation of experimentally induced presleep experiences to dreams. *Journal of the American Psychoanalytic Association, 13*, 819–849.

Witkin, H. & Lewis, H. (Eds.) (1967). *Experimental studies in dreaming*. New York: Random House.

Witkin, H., Lewis, H., Hertzman, M., Machover, K., Meissner, P., & Wapner, J. (1954). *Personality through perception*. New York: Harper & Row.

Witkin, H., Dyk, R., Goodenough, D., Faterson, H., & Karp, S. (1962). *Psychological differentiation.* New York: Wiley.

Wolchik, S., Beggs, V., Wincze, J., Sakheim, D., Barlow, D., & Mavissakalian, M. (1980). The effect of emotional arousal on subsequent sexual arousal in men. *Journal of Abnormal and Social Psychology, 89,* 595–599.

Wolff, P. (1960). The developmental psychologies of Jean Piaget and psychoanalysis. *Psychological Issues* Monograph Series (Vol. 2, No. 5) 2, Monograph No. 5.

Wolff, P. (1969). The natural history of crying and other vocalization in early infancy. In B. M. Foss (Ed.), *Determinants of infant behaviors.* London: Methuen.

Zajonc, R. (1980). Feeling and thinking. *American Psychologist, 35,* 151–175.

Zimmerman, W. (1967). *Psychological and physiological differences between "light" and "deep" sleepers.* Paper presented at the meeting of the Association for the Psychophysiological Study of Sleep, Santa Monica.

Index

229